NOW HEAL THIS...

Eating to Save Your Life.

A Cookbook

Author
Tina Ellerby

Co-Author
Cathleen Seaquist

Grain–free, Gluten–free, Sugar–free Eating

ISBN: 098376350X
ISBN-13: 9780983763505

Library of Congress Control Number: 2013950320
2WellnessNow, L.L.P.
Stuart, Florida

.

PUBLISHER'S NOTE
Neither the publisher nor the authors are engaged in rendering professional advice or services to the individual reader. The dietary suggestions, programs, recipes, resources, ideas, and procedures contained in this book are not intended as a substitute for consulting a health care professional. Consultation with your health practitioner where appropriate, is advised. The advice and strategies contained herein may not be suitable for your situation. The publisher and authors are not responsible for your specific health or allergy needs that may require medical supervision, for any adverse reactions to the recipes or products contained or referred to in this book, or for any loss or damage arising or allegedly arising, from any information or suggestions in this book. Every attempt has been made by the authors and publisher of this book to provide accurate telephone numbers and internet addresses as of the time of publication, neither party assume any responsibility for errors, or changes that occur after publication.

This recipe book is proudly made in the United States of America.

2WellnessNow is a registered L.L.P., operating in the state of Florida.
Visit us at 2WellnessNow.com or follow us on:
FACEBOOK, TWITTER, and PINTEREST at NOW HEAL THIS.

DEDICATION

To God,
for placing me upon this path to wellness.

To Dr. Michael Balas,
there are no words
to adequately express my thanks.
God has blessed you with a true gift.
I owe *you* my life,
but thank *Him* for it every day.

CONTENTS

OFF TO WELLNESS   vii

INTRODUCTION   xi

BASICS   1

BEVERAGES   29

RISE 'N SHINE   43

ON-THE-GO   59

APPETIZERS   77

SOUPS   97

SALADS   111

VEGGIES   125

ENTRÉES   144

DESSERTS   186

"GO-TO" GUIDE   219

TESTIMONIALS   224

INDEX   227

ABOUT THE AUTHORS   230

"The doctor of the future
will give no medicine,
but will interest his patients
in the care of the human frame,
in a proper diet,
and in the cause and
prevention of disease."

Thomas Edison
U.S. Inventor
1847 – 1931

OFF TO WELLNESS

One of the key factors in helping heal or maintain health is controlling the foods you eat. Adhering to a low-glycemic eating plan is the single most important thing we should ALL do to improve health. Why? Because eating sugars, grains, and starches [including root vegetables (yes, even carrots), or popular favorites like peas, and corn] make our blood sugar levels spike high, which in turn make our bodies secrete insulin to help lower sugar levels. This repetitive pattern of sugar spiking and lowering is the catalyst for ill-health, and the breeding ground for many diseases. So, the goal for us should be to avoid sugar spikes, and keep our blood sugars on an even keel.

A low-glycemic eating plan is one that eliminates grains and sugars. Elimination of grains and high-carbohydrate foods would include, but not be limited to, anything made from wheat, rice, corn, oats, barley, rye, or any "healthy" whole grain (including that organic, locally grown, ground, and fresh-baked 12-grain bread). Elimination of sugars would include, but not be limited to: table sugar, molasses, honey, cane sugar, cane juice, high-fructose corn syrup (HFCS), corn syrup, maple syrup, dextrose, sucrose, fructose (and almost any other ingredient that ends with an "ose"). So...step away from the fruit, unless it's berries or Granny Smith apples (organic, of course).

Do you want the realization of improvement in your physical health to be *easy*, or do you want it to be the *best* it can be? The choice is yours.

It is equally important on your path to wellness for you to eliminate as many toxins (ingested, inhaled, or absorbed) as possible. There are many toxic exposures you may choose to eliminate, if you are aware that they exist.

- Did you know that your antiperspirant/deodorant has been *leeching aluminum into your bloodstream* for all the years you've been using it?

- Did you know that cooking with your food wrapped in aluminum foil or in metal pots and pans (including those that are Teflon coated), *exposes your entire family to chemical and heavy metal toxicity?*

- Fluoride (an extremely toxic heavy metal) exists in your tap water, toothpaste, and mouthwash. It is typically *not removed* even when you filter your water.

- Two of the most toxic ingredients in health care products are *parabens* and *sulfates*. These are some of the ingredients in your *makeup, bubble bath products* (yes, even your child's), *facial creams,* and even your husband's *body wash* (to name a few). Our bodies absorb everything we apply to our skin. We should think twice before applying *anything* to it. After all, it is the *largest organ* of our body.

- You know to be careful of the sun's UV rays, but did you know that most of your *suntan lotions are laden with toxic chemicals,* which are absorbed by your skin?

- Chlorine is a toxic chemical, often added to our *water supplies,* and most often used in our *pools* and *hot tubs.* Exposure to it should be eliminated.

- Mercury fillings (amalgams), *leech mercury every day* into our bodies. Consideration should be given to abatement of amalgams to eliminate this horrible source of heavy metal toxicity.

- Eliminate food that is considered to be GMO (genetically modified), in particular soy beans and soy products. Soy sauce (wheat-free varieties manufactured outside of the US) are considered safe for consumption as they are fermented. Soy product elimination will cause you to omit 85% of the processed food you purchase. Read your labels, and put your best cooking aprons on!

- Overuse of prescription drugs, particularly steroids and antibiotics, cause *iatrogenic diseases* and *disorders* (diseases or disorders caused by medical treatment or advice from physicians, pharmacists, etc., or adverse side effects, or complications from, drugs or therapies given). Work with your holistic healer to understand the necessity, as well as the side effects expected, from any prescription or over-the-counter medicine, as well as your supplements.

- Chemical sweeteners, as well as chemical cleaners, bombard your body with neurotoxins. Danger! Danger! Avoid these poisons.

We encourage you to read...read...read. And when you're done, read some more. Go to your holistic practitioner with any questions. We hope you get tired, of being sick and tired.

Remember, the *speed* at which your body recovers, and the *degree* to which it recovers, depends greatly on you and the choices you *do* or *do not* make.

Fight for your health. No one else will.

INTRODUCTION

Have you ever gotten so desperately sick, that you'd try *anything* to feel better? That's where I found myself in the early winter of 2007. For decades I had been told by my doctors and specialists (including an internist, cardiologist, endocrinologist, rheumatologist, and pulmonologist), that in order to get healthy I needed to eat a "low fat" diet inclusive of "whole grain" foods. I did *just* that. I continued to get sick. Medications were added and doses "tweaked," as my body succumbed to a host of medical issues. I dutifully took *every* pill, had *every* test, and followed *every* recommendation. I became sicker.

In November of 2007, I was treated at a local emergency room for difficulty breathing, heart palpitations, and blood pressure spikes. They gave me their best diagnosis. "It's your gall bladder." The only problem with that diagnosis was that I had my gall bladder removed 15 years prior. Their second diagnosis; I was having a "heart" issue. Not a far reach, as I had been treated for almost two decades as an overweight diabetic with discoid lupus, asthma, COPD, heart arrhythmias, high cholesterol, and high blood pressure. Though they seemed confident that my heart was the "issue" their tests showed nothing. They decided that raising my blood pressure medication would make everything go away. The look of concern in my husband's eyes made me incredibly sad. I left the hospital with no explanations, more medications, and the sickening feeling that I was on the fast-track to dying.

Enter, Dr. Michael Balas, a chiropractor. A friend highly recommended him as an "alternative" doctor, and suggested I make an appointment. I was desperate. I made the call and begged Dr. Balas to see me at his earliest convenience. I knew that unless something in my life drastically changed, my medications were going to kill me, and I was going to let them. I felt 96, and more than ready to meet my Maker, at the ripe old age of...48.

Dr. Balas took everything I *knew* to be *true*, and threw it out the window. I sat in front of him desperate and broken. I was willing to try *anything*. And so I did. I couldn't give you one logical reason why I chose to listen to him that day. After all, I had been an Advanced Emergency Medical Technician for years in my younger days. I was familiar with the medical field, its doctors, hospitals, tests, and teachings. I had been told what to do, what to eat, and what was right for me and my body. I was fairly sure that everything Dr. B. was suggesting was going to kill me, faster. A small voice inside me asked- *what do you have to lose?*

I had never questioned the knowledge I had gathered from my doctors and nutritionists for decades. I assumed it was all true. I heard the same things over and over again. I did have some concerns that Dr. B. was a quack (with a capital "Q"), when I heard him rattle off the list of food he wanted me to start eating. But, desperate times, dictated desperate measures. I decided to follow his suggestions. Not only was he *correct*, but I have come to find that much of what he passed along is not new science, technology, or thinking. As hard as it is to believe, a huge part of helping my body heal from disease started with choosing the right foods. As a society, we have been directed by scientific, political, and pharmaceutical influences, to believe that eating all the *wrong* foods is somehow *right* for our health. Overcoming the belief that "popular or common" medical treatments were "normal or healthy" for me, was my biggest challenge.

Dr. B. didn't lecture me. He taught me. He carefully explained the physiology of our body's systems, and how they work together for *health* -- or many times (as in my case), *DIS-EASE*. He explained the importance, for all of mankind, to remove as many toxic challenges to their bodies as possible. He encouraged me to eliminate grains, sugars, chemical sweeteners, and all soy products. *I could do that! Couldn't I?*

That afternoon, Friday, January 18, 2008, I started eating the way Dr. B. had suggested. On Sunday, January 20th, only two days later, I was no longer taking three of my 13 medications. I had started that weekend as an insulin-injecting diabetic. I ended that weekend, as a non-insulin injecting diabetic. I was ecstatic. I hated needles, and in two days time had eliminated my need for three separate injections, three times a day- that I had required for *years* prior. A few days later, it hit me. My being better wasn't just a fluke! It had everything to do with the food I was putting in my mouth. 40% of my food is protein, 30% of my food is saturated animal fat, and 30% of my food is carbohydrates (from non-root vegetables, and limited fruit).

My rewards were *immediate*. Today, I jokingly tell Dr. B., that it's much harder to be healthy than it is to be sick, because I have to *choose* it- *every day,* and at *every meal.*

It meant I eliminated refined flours, all carbohydrates (except for specific vegetables), all sugars (except for berries), all chemical sweeteners, and all soy products.

"Oh," I hear you say…"is that ALL?" Hard? You bet it was hard! But, nothing is impossible if you set your mind to it. I don't understand why some people would look at this eating plan and see it as *denying* themselves something. I see at it as *rewarding* myself with *everything.*

It is my belief, that God has blessed Dr. Balas with the gift of healing and teaching. I am humbled at the opportunity to have been placed in his path. It is also my belief that God designed our bodies to be able to fight disease, ALL disease.

Why did I write this cookbook, when there are a "bazillion" other cookbooks on the market? The answer is simple. I want to be an encourager in the world of low-glycemic, non-insulin spiking eating plans that are catalysts for good health in ALL people, not just diabetics. I want to encourage readers to seek and gain knowledge about how their body systems are actually designed to function, versus how they are currently functioning; to never be afraid to ask questions about their health; and to learn to just say, "No," if they don't feel satisfied with the answers they are getting from any source, including medical professionals. I want to encourage readers to seek holistic healers (chiropractors, naturopaths, applied kinesiologists, homeopaths), anyone who believes that the approach to illness does not require drugs or surgery. I would direct you specifically to those who are familiar with low-glycemic eating plans and their effects on overall health. It didn't hurt, that my doctor, Doctor B. is also a teacher of anatomy and physiology.

Change the way you think. Change the way you eat. Crave knowledge. Don't just settle for answers. Be an informed decision maker.

Your road to wellness starts now. The choice is yours.

Tina Ellerby
Author

Daily posts for living well in a low-glycemic,
grain-free, sugar-free, gluten-free world,
may be found on:

FACEBOOK, as NOW HEAL THIS

Also follow us on
TWITTER and PINTEREST

Visit our website at 2wellnessnow.com
for recipe ideas, testimonials, and information to help guide you
through a grain-free, sugar-free, and gluten-free lifestyle

A.W.E. (A.lternate W.ay of E.ating)
AWE's are listed at the bottom of each recipe.

These represent changes to either an ingredient, or the serving or preparation techniques, and are meant to inspire you.

FACT
A fact is noted at the bottom of each recipe to help expand your overall knowledge.

We believe that knowledge is the key to health.

<u>TERMS USED IN THIS BOOK:</u>

GREASED: we are referring to greasing a pan with COCONUT OIL (pg. 219) up to 350 degrees OR with GRAPE SEED OIL (pg. 220), for temperatures 350 and higher.

WATER: we mean filtered water

SALT: we mean FINE SEA SALT not iodized table salt

PEPPER: we mean FRESHLY GROUND BLACK PEPPER

COCONUT: we mean UNSWEETENED varieties

(fresh or dried, flaked, shredded, or finely grated)

COCOA: we mean UNSWEETENED COCOA POWDER

CHOCOLATE: (milk or dark) we are referring to MALITOL-SWEETENED, commercially available chocolate bars, unless stated otherwise (pg. 219).

BAKING POWDER: we mean ALUMINUM-FREE varieties

DOUBLE BOILER: we mean a non-direct heat source, usually a bowl placed over a smaller saucepan filled with water, over medium high heat.

MILK: we mean ORGANIC (Grass-fed, Raw where allowable) WHOLE MILK

PROTEINS: we mean ORGANIC, GRASS-FED varieties where possible

SAUSAGE: we mean SUGAR and WHEAT-FREE varieties

BACON: we refer to NITRATE-FREE bacon

SALAMI/PEPPERONI: should be suspect for wheat and/or sugar influences

BUTTER: we refer to SALTED ORGANIC or RAW BUTTER

CHICKEN BROTH: we refer to ORGANIC varieties with NO SUGAR ADDED, or homemade

If a particular dish size is not mentioned in a recipe, then the size of the dish you choose, should not significantly affect cooking time.

BASICS

- **Romano Rounds**
- **Parmesan Crispers**
- **"Faux" Crackers**
- **Cheddary Bites**
- **A Tisket...A Biscuit**
- **Mayonnaise**
- **Ketchup**
- **Cucumber Yogurt Sauce**
- **No Skimpin' Shrimpin'**
  (Cocktail Sauce)
- **Dippy Fishy**
  (Tartar Sauce)
- **Herb Butter**
- **Cheese-y Please-y**
  (Cheese Sauce)
- **Holler for Hollandaise**
- **Roasted Garlic 'N Horseradish Sauce**

- **There's 'Shroom for Steak**
  (Steak Sauce)
- **Churri — Slurry**
  (Chimichurri Sauce)
- *Presto*...Pesto!
- **Chicken Gravy**
- **Vinegary BBQ Sauce**
- **"Matoey" BBQ Sauce**
- **"Mato" Sauce**
- **White 'N Fluffy Spread**
- **"Faux" Brown Sugar**
- **Granny's Applesauce**
- **Granny's Crannies**
  (Chunky Cranberry Sauce)
- **Oh, Dough!**
- **Toasted Pecan Crust**

Building Basics
Building Blocks for Healthy Choices

"Good health, and good sense,
are two of life's greatest blessings."

Publilius Syrus
Latin Writer
1st Century, B.C.

ROMANO ROUNDS
(dipping chips, or salad toppers)

A handful of Romano cheese, finely shredded

Into a small (heated but dry) ceramic-lined frying pan, place the Romano cheese. Allow it to melt. Once cheese has lightly browned, flip and continue cooking until the second side has browned. Cool on wire rack completely before breaking it into pieces.

Don't you love being cheesy?

A.W.E. – *while cheese is warm, cut it into pie shaped dipping chips using a pizza wheel, or a pair of kitchen scissors*

FACT: *Romano cheese may be frozen if cut into ½ lb. chunks. Freeze in airtight containers. Thaw in refrigerator. Use immediately once defrosted.*

PARMESAN CRISPERS
(dipping chips, or salad toppers)

Preheat oven to 375 degrees
1-½ cups parmesan cheese, grated
2 tsps. almond flour
1 tsp. coconut flour
1 to 2 tsps. minced herbs or spices of your choice
2 parchment lined baking sheets

Mix all ingredients. Drop 1-½ Tablespoons of cheese onto parchment paper, 3" apart. Flatten cheese using the back of the spoon. Bake in a single layer (one baking sheet at a time), on the middle rack of oven, 7 to 9 minutes, or until golden. Cool on wire rack.

Finger licking good.

A.W.E. – *ADD half parmesan and half asiago cheeses*

FACT: *A vegetable peeler "shaves" parmesan cheese for salads, or garnishes.*

"FAUX" CRACKERS

Think differently.
When serving a cheese platter, consider "faux" crackers, too.

Don't default to celery sticks.

TRY USING:

* Walnut halves, flat side up
(great topped with cream cheese, and a sliced olive)
* Individual endive leaves
* Slices of granny smith apples
* Pork rinds
* Small tomatoes, cored
* Thick slices of pepperoni or salami, raw or baked
* Cucumber rounds (instead of just "spears")
english cucumbers have less seeds and are not as wet
* Cucumber boats.
Peel cucumber. Cut width-wise making ½" slices.
Use a melon-baller, removing seeds but not cutting all the way through.
Fill the center with your favorite spread.

May the FAUX be with you.

A.W.E. *– oven bake slices of pepperoni, OR salami, to "crisp" them up*

FACT: *To achieve optimal health, you should be concerned
about controlling your blood sugar levels and eliminating insulin spikes.
Eating grain and sugar – free accomplishes this without a second thought.*

CHEDDARY BITES

2-¼ cups almond flour
¼ cup chickpea flour
1-½ cups cheddar cheese, finely grated
1 tsp. guar gum (pg. 220)
½ tsp. baking soda
¼ tsp. sea salt
2 eggs
1 egg white
3 Tbsps. grape seed oil
extra sea salt for topping
parchment paper & 3 large baking sheets
(or two and some patience)

Preheat oven to 350 degrees

Cut four sheets of parchment paper the size of your baking sheets. In a bowl combine: almond flour, chickpea flour, cheddar cheese, guar gum, baking soda, and ¼ tsp. salt. In a small, second bowl, mix eggs, egg white, and grape seed oil, whisking well. Mix wet ingredients into dry and combine. Divide dough into 3 even portions. Place 1 piece of dough in between two pieces of parchment, and roll as thinly as possible. Remove top piece of parchment paper, and place the rolled out dough, onto the cookie sheet. Repeat for remaining portions of dough, set aside until ready to bake. Use a pizza cutter or knife, cut dough into desired cracker size. Poke dough with the tines of a fork, and then sprinkle dough with salt. Bake crackers one baking sheet at a time, for 15 to 18 minutes, or until edges turn light brown. Rescore crackers immediately upon removal from oven. Transfer parchment with crackers to a cooling rack. Allow crackers to cool completely, before storing in an airtight container.

We love crumbs.

A.W.E. – *ADD a little "zing" of your choosing...tabasco, horseradish, OR cayenne pepper*

FACT: *Grape seed oil has a light taste, a smoke point of about 485 degrees, and is a non-hydrogenated.*

A Tisket...A BISCUIT

2-¼ cups almond flour
¼ cup chickpea flour
1 Tbsp. coconut flour
3 Tbsps. coconut oil, melted (no substitutions)
2 tsps. guar gum (pg. 220)
¼ tsp. sea salt
1 Tbsp. xylitol sweetener
1-½ tsps. baking powder
2 eggs
½ cup + 2 Tbsps. heavy cream
2 Tbsps. whole milk

Preheat oven to 400 degrees

SIFT almond flour, and chickpea flour into a large bowl, and add coconut oil, mixing until well combined. Mix in guar gum, salt, xylitol, and baking powder. Add eggs and mix well. Add heavy cream, and milk. Once mixed, allow dough to sit for five minutes. Place heaping tablespoons of dough onto parchment lined baking sheet. Bake 13 to 15 minutes (depending on size of biscuit), until a hint of brown appears on top edges.

Share.

A.W.E. – *ADD your favorite herbs.*
OR – try *combinations such as:*
sun-dried tomato and feta cheese
OR – lemon and thyme
OR – use them to make your SANDWICH for lunch time

FACT: *Guar gum improves the texture,
and shelf life of baked goods, and is popular in gluten-free recipes.*

MAYONNAISE

2 large eggs
1 tsp. white vinegar
1 tsp. fresh lemon juice
⅛ tsp. xylitol sweetener, finely ground
(in a coffee bean grinder)
½ tsp. sea salt
¼ tsp. onion powder
¼ tsp. dijon mustard
¼ tsp. hot sauce
1 cup grape seed oil

In a medium-size mixing bowl add all ingredients EXCEPT for oil. Use the whisk attachment of an electric mixer to combine well (about ten seconds) on high speed. Leaving whisk on, add the oil to the egg mixture in a slow, thin, steady stream. Beat until thick and creamy. Add extra vinegar for tartness, or xylitol for sweetness, to personal taste. If mayonnaise is too thick to your liking, add water, 1 tsp. at a time, until desired thickness is achieved. Refrigerate in an air-tight container before serving. Mayonnaise will also thicken as it chills. Remember to date your container, this homemade variety will last about 3 day.

A little dab'll do it.

A.W.E. – *FLAVOR YOUR MAYO:*
1 cup mayo; 2 cloves garlic, minced;
8 fresh basil leaves chopped; s&p
OR – 1 cup mayo; 3 tsps. horseradish; 8 fresh tarragon leaves, chopped; s&p
OR – 1 cup mayo; 2 Tbsps. fresh dill, chopped; zest of ½ lemon; s&p
OR – 1 cup mayo; 1 tsp chipotle powder; ½ shallot, minced; s&p

FACT: *Consisting of mostly egg yolks, homemade mayonnaise usually appears more yellow in color than store-bought mayonnaise. To lighten its appearance, you may add a little more lemon juice.*

KETCHUP

1 can tomato puree (28 oz.)
2 Tbsps. onion powder
¼ cup xylitol sweetener
½ cup lemon juice
¾ tsp. sea salt
¼ tsp. dry mustard
⅛ tsp. ground ginger
⅛ tsp. garlic powder
⅛ tsp. cayenne red pepper
⅛ tsp. ground allspice
1 pinch ground cloves (or 2 clove heads, crushed)
1 pinch cinnamon

Place all ingredients into a medium pot. Bring to a boil, uncovered. Immediately upon boiling, reduce to simmer. Cover and cook for 1-½ hours, stirring occasionally. Uncover and cook an additional 45 minutes before adjusting flavors (xylitol for sweetness, or lemon juice for tartness), to personal taste. Continue simmering uncovered, to desired consistency. This may take up to 4 more hours. Remove from heat and cool completely. Store in an airtight container in refrigerator, or freeze for future use. Allow ketchup to set-up for 24 hours prior to first use. Date your containers, this ketchup has about a three week shelf life.

Everything's better with ketchup.

A.W.E. – *for a spicy version ADD a little chipotle, or chili powder
OR – use green tomatoes*

FACT: *Cayenne pepper is a potent stimulant to
the entire body, and aids in digestion.
It has been used to relieve pain and inflammation.*

CUCUMBER YOGURT SAUCE

2 seedless cucumbers
1 cup plain greek yogurt
1 cup sour cream
1 tsp. lemon juice
2 tsps. chopped mixed herbs (dill, parsley, basil, etc.)
sea salt & freshly ground black pepper

Peel cucumbers, and grate finely into a mixing bowl. Add yogurt, sour cream, lemon juice and herbs, mixing well. Season with salt and pepper to personal taste. Refrigerate a minimum of two hours prior to serving.

Cool your cukes!

A.W.E. – *use fresh, chopped garlic, dill,
and shallots in place of mixed herbs
OR – use fresh chopped mint with lemon peel*

FACT: *Greek style yogurt is thicker than traditional yogurt,
with more protein per serving.*

CUCUMBER TIDBIT

- The State of Florida provides about one third of our national supply of cucumbers. California, New Jersey, and New York are also large producers.

NO SKIMPIN' SHRIMPIN'
Cocktail Sauce

1 cup Ketchup (pg. 8)
1 heaping Tbsp. prepared horseradish
(more, or less, to personal taste)
freshly ground black pepper

Mix all ingredients together until well combined. Store in an air tight container and refrigerate. Date your container. Serve chilled.

Where's the shrimp?

A.W.E. – *ADD a little tabasco sauce OR chili powder*

FACT: *In Iceland, sour cream is considered essential to cocktail sauce.*

DIPPY FISHY
Tartar Sauce

1-½ cups Mayonnaise (pg. 7)
1 medium-size sour pickle, diced
4 shallots, peeled, finely diced
1 Tbsp. fresh parsley, finely chopped
1 Tbsp. dried tarragon
1 tsp. fresh lemon juice
sea salt and freshly ground black pepper

Place mayonnaise, pickle, shallots, parsley, tarragon, and lime juice into a small bowl, whisking until well combined. Add salt and pepper to personal taste. Chill before use. Store in a dated, airtight container.

Here fishy, fishy, fishy.

A.W.E. – *use capers with, or instead of, sour pickle*

FACT: *The caper bush has rounded, fleshy leaves, with pinkish-white flowers. Capers are its edible flower buds.*

HERB BUTTER

1 stick salted butter, room temperature
6 fresh chives, minced
1-½ Tbsps. fresh thyme, minced
1-½ Tbsps. fresh rosemary, minced
sea salt and freshly ground black pepper to taste

Mix all ingredients well. Roll herbed butter into a log shape using a piece of parchment paper. Freeze for one hour, or refrigerate for several hours, before use. Slice *across* tube to form "pats" of butter.

A.W.E. – *ADD garlic, and replace the thyme & rosemary with basil*

FACT: *Do not accept margarine or "imitation" butter
substitutes in your healthy eating plan.
Choose butter over "hydrogenated"
or "partially hydrogenated" alternatives.*

USE YOUR IMAGINATION
for
COMPOUND BUTTER COMBINATIONS

Rosemary, parmesan cheese, garlic, s&p
Garlic & dill, s&p
Fresh rosemary, roasted garlic, s&p
Parsley, capers, lemon zest, s&p
Red pepper, oregano, s&p
Tarragon, lime juice, s&p
Chipotle, lime, s&p
Dijon mustard, garlic, thyme, s&p
Blue Cheese, chive (or scallion), s&p
Porcini mushrooms, s&p
Basil, cilantro, s&p

Endless possibilities...

CHEESE-Y PLEASE-Y
Cheese Sauce

1 cup heavy cream
1 cup sharp cheddar cheese, diced
1 cup mozzarella cheese
2 Tbsps. butter
2 cloves fresh garlic, smashed and chopped
1 tsp. mustard
1 tsp. sea salt

Melt all ingredients in the top of a double boiler, over medium heat. Add all ingredients to top pot. Stir constantly until cheese sauce is smooth. Serve immediately.

Geeez...CHEESE!!

A.W.E. – *ADD ½ cup salsa*
OR – *OMIT mustard and ADD 1 tsp. horseradish, and/or chopped, fresh rosemary*

FACT: *Mozzarella Cheese is typically made with either pasteurized, or unpasteurized cow's milk, or domesticated water buffalo milk.*

HOLLER for HOLLANDAISE Sauce

*note: this recipe makes about 1 cup

6 Tbsps. unsalted butter, softened
3 egg yolks
¼ cup boiling water
1 tsp. fresh lemon juice
pinch cayenne pepper
sea salt

In a double boiler (or heat-proof bowl over, but not touching, simmering water), add butter and egg yolks whisking constantly. Add the ¼ cup of boiling water slowly while continuing to whisk until the mixture reaches 160 degrees or starts to thicken. This should take 8 to 10 minutes. Remove from heat, and add lemon, cayenne pepper, and salt to personal taste. Serve immediately over things like eggs, steak, crab, or veggies. Your choice.

Over anything.

A.W.E. *– use a little tarragon vinegar if you don't have lemon juice*

FACT: *Hollandaise is one of the five basic sauces
in French Cuisine.
It is believed to have been named, and designed,
for the King of the Netherlands, when he visited France,
to mimic a Dutch sauce he enjoyed.*

ROASTED GARLIC 'N HORSERADISH SAUCE

1-½ cups sour cream
½ cup Mayonnaise (pg. 7)
3 Tbsps. fresh horseradish
sea salt and freshly ground black pepper
1 entire head of garlic, roasted

Preheat oven to 400 degrees

To roast garlic, cut off the top of the entire head, leaving white paper skin on the outside of the bulb. Add pats of butter, salt, and pepper to the cut top. Wrap garlic in parchment lined aluminum foil, making a tent. Seal the top of the foil by crimping it. Bake at 400 degrees, for 30 to 35 minutes. Once head has cooled, the garlic cloves will easily squeeze out of their skins. Mash cloves and mix all ingredients in a bowl. Store in an airtight container for a few days.

Make your radish...horse.

A.W.E. – *ADD diced scallions, or chives*
OR – ADD scallions, bacon and shredded cheddar cheese

FACT: *Garlic is related to the leek, and the onion.*
Garlic contains powerful nutrients that help fight disease.
Roasting is a common method of preparation, giving this typically
pungent food a milder, sweeter taste.

THERE's 'SHROOM FOR STEAK
(Steak Sauce. A Treat for Meat)

*this recipe requires making Ketchup (pg. 8)
before preparation.

2 cups ketchup
1 can sliced mushrooms
3 Tbsps. horseradish
4 oz. butter
sea salt and freshly ground black pepper to taste

Heat all ingredients in a saucepan on low, until heated through. Use immediately or refrigerate in an airtight container.

Where's the beef?

A.W.E. – *ADD some sautéed onions, shallots, or leeks*
OR – try it as a salad dressing (sounds weird, tastes great) by
ADDING some crumbled blue cheese

FACT: *Mushrooms are neither animal, nor plant, but FUNGUS.*
The part of the fungus that we see, and eat, is actually only
the fruit of the organism itself.

PEPPER TIDBITS

• Pepper is the number one selling spice in America.

• Pepper comes in many colors such as green, black, red, and white, but all come from the same plant. The color is related to how ripe it is when harvested, as well as the way it is processed.

CHURRI – SLURRY
(Chimichurri Sauce)

8 cloves fresh garlic, chopped
1-½ cups olive oil
2 small shallots, chopped
1-½ cups cilantro
½ tsp. crushed red pepper
juice of 4 limes
sea salt to taste

Put all ingredients except for oil, into a food processor/blender. Pulse ingredients while adding oil in three portions. DO NOT OVER BLEND. *The consistency should be thicker than a puree.* Allow to sit room temperature, for *2 hours* before serving.

Hurry up 'n make the "churri"!

A.W.E. – *OMIT cilantro and ADD parsley*
AND substitute red wine vinegar for lime juice
OR – ADD a little oregano

FACT: *Shallots are available fresh whole, chopped, or dried.*
Store them in a cool, dry place for at least two months.
Shallots may be frozen, but lose their crunch after thawing.
Don't buy sprouting shallots (an indication of age).
Young, small shallots, have a milder flavor than larger ones.

*PRESTO...*PESTO!

2 cups fresh basil leaves, packed
½ cup parmesan or romano cheese, freshly grated
⅓ cup pine nuts
3 cloves fresh garlic
½ cup extra virgin olive oil
sea salt and freshly ground black pepper
food processor, or blender

Place basil and pine nuts into food processor/blender. Pulse a few times, but do not puree. Add garlic. Pulse a few times again. Now, turn processor/blender on constant low, adding olive oil in a continuous stream. When oil is incorporated, stop mixing. Add cheese. Use a pulsing action to incorporate. Pour into a bowl. Add salt and pepper to taste, stirring well. Serve. Store (or freeze), in dated air-tight containers.

We love green food.

A.W.E. – *substitute walnuts for pine nuts*
OR – cut basil in half, and ADD 8 oz. of roasted red bell pepper

FACT: *The basil plant is an easy one to grow,*
which makes it one of the most popular among home chefs.
Basil is a member of the Mint family.

CHICKEN GRAVY

1 small yellow onion (or ½ medium onion), finely chopped
3 Tbsps. butter
4 cloves fresh garlic, minced
2 Tbsps. chickpea flour
1 cup heavy cream
1 cup chicken broth
1 tsp. dried sage
½ tsp. sea salt
¼ tsp. freshly ground black pepper

In a saucepan, melt butter over medium heat. Sauté onion and garlic until soft and lightly browned (6 to 8 minutes). Add chickpea flour, stirring constantly for about 1 minute. Whisk in chicken broth, sage, salt and pepper. Stir occasionally while bringing to boil. Once boiling, reduce heat and stir continually until desired thickness. Serve immediately.

Crave-e, gravy.

A.W.E. – *OMIT sage and ADD 1 tsp. curry powder*
OR – use coconut milk in place of heavy cream

FACT: *GRAVY is commonly referred to as the liquid part of a dish. There's Chocolate gravy, Cream gravy, Egg gravy, Giblet gravy, Onion gravy, Spiced gravy, Tomato gravy, Vegetable gravy, and White gravy...to name a few.*

VINEGARY BBQ SAUCE

1 cup apple cider vinegar
2 Tbsps. sea salt
1 Tbsp. "Faux" Brown Sugar (pg. 23)
1 tsp. cayenne pepper
1 tsp. crushed red pepper

Combine all ingredients in a small pot. Cook uncovered, on medium heat, until dissolved. Serve warm, or room temperature.

Yes, please.

A.W.E. – *OMIT cayenne & crushed red pepper,*
and ADD 1 Tbsp. chili powder, 1 tsp. paprika, and 1-½ tsps. dry mustard

FACT: *BBQ sauces come in many different styles*
and use many different bases in recipes.
These bases include: vinegar and pepper; tomato sauce;
ketchup; mustard; as well as dry rubs.
There is no such thing as "wrong."
Find your favorite flavors and build on them.

"MATOEY" BBQ SAUCE

1 cup Ketchup (pg. 8)
½ tsp. sea salt
1 tsp. spicy brown mustard
2 Tbsps. lemon juice
2 Tbsps. apple cider vinegar
½ medium onion, chopped
1 Tbsp. butter
2 celery stalks (with green leafy tops), finely chopped
2 Tbsps. xylitol sweetener
¼ to ½ tsp. cayenne pepper (depending on how "hot" you want it)

Sauté celery & onion in butter, until onions are translucent. Add all other ingredients and stir. Simmer on low heat for a minimum of 20 minutes (if you have time- the longer it cooks, the better it gets). Yields enough for 1 lb. of meat.

Makes you want to eat your fingers !

A.W.E. – *ADD 2 cloves of fresh garlic, minced*

FACT: *Vinegar has been shown to help lower blood sugar levels.*
Go easy using vinegars in any of your recipes
if you suffer with mold sensitivities.

"MATO" SAUCE

2 Tbsps. coconut oil
2 Tbsps. butter
1 large yellow onion, chopped
4 cloves garlic, pressed or minced
1 can tomato puree (28 oz.)
1 cup water
1-½ tsps. sea salt
2 Tbsps. tomato paste
1 tsp. dried marjoram
½ tsp. freshly ground black pepper
2 cans tomato sauce (15 oz. - no sugar added)
2 Tbsps. dried parsley
1-½ Tbsps. dried oregano
2 tsps. dried basil
1 bay leaf

Heat butter and coconut oil in large skillet and sauté onion and garlic over medium heat until tender. Add all remaining ingredients, and simmer for at least one hour. *Remember, the flavor is developed in the simmering. The longer it cooks, the better it is.* Sauce may be frozen in airtight containers for future use.

Spoon-dipping encouraged.

A.W.E. – *ADD cooked ground beef*
OR – ADD crushed red pepper for some spice
OR – ADD turmeric for a zesty kick
OR – if you like it chunky- OMIT 2 cans tomato sauce and
ADD 2 cans (15 oz.) or 1 can (28 oz.) of crushed tomatoes

FACT: *Marjoram may be substituted for oregano in equal*
proportions in recipes, and vice-versa.
Marjoram has a mild oregano-like taste.
A little goes a long way.

WHITE 'N FLUFFY SPREAD

*** note: this recipe requires lengthy refrigeration before use,
and uses egg whites that are not cooked.*

1 packet non-flavored gelatin
½ cup filtered water
1-½ cups heavy cream
2 tsps. vanilla extract
pinch of sea salt
** 4 egg whites
6 Tbsps. xylitol sweetener,
(finely ground in a coffee bean grinder)

In a small bowl, soak gelatin in water, and set it aside. In a heavy-bottomed saucepan over low heat, stirring often, bring the cream to just before a boil. Remove from heat. Add gelatin, vanilla, and salt. Stir continually until the gelatin is completely dissolved. Stir mixture occasionally as it completely cools. This will take about 1-½ hours. Once mixture has completely cooled, in a medium bowl mix egg whites until soft-peaked. Add xylitol, one tablespoon at a time, mixing well until all is incorporated. Stir chilled gelatin mixture into the egg whites in four portions, whisking well between each addition. Store in an airtight container and refrigerate. Spread will thicken as it chills. This is great spread on slices of granny smith apples with some of your favorite nut butter.

Sweet. Treat.
Good enough to eat (on anything).

A.W.E. *– sprinkle toasted coconut OR chopped nuts on top*

FACT: *The white of an egg is composed of 90% water and 10% protein.*

"FAUX" BROWN SUGAR

1 cup xylitol sweetener
1 tsp. maple extract
1 tsp. vanilla extract
½ tsp. ground cinnamon
1 Tbsp. Nature's Hollow sugar-free honey

Combine all ingredients in a bowl, stirring well. Allow mixture to sit for 15 minutes, before use in a recipe.

Sugar. Dah-dah, dah-dah, dah-dah...

A.W.E. – *OMIT cinnamon*
*OR – use Granulated Coconut Nectar as a non-chemical substitute for brown sugar in baking. It has a much higher glycemic index,
and should be used sparingly*

FACT: *Xylitol is well documented in its ability to aid people
with improved oral health.*

CINNAMON TIDBITS

- Cinnamon is a tree, and its bark is used to make the spice. Cinnamalehyde is the compound in the bark that gives cinnamon its scent and flavor.

- Cinnamon contains manganese, fiber, iron, and calcium.

- The best cinnamon is Ceylon cinnamon from Sri Lanka.

GRANNY'S APPLESAUCE

8 granny smith apples, peeled, cored (4 finely diced, 4 cubed)
¾ cup water
⅛ tsp. sea salt
⅛ tsp. vanilla extract
1-½ tsps. ground cinnamon
½ cup xylitol sweetener

Over medium heat, place all ingredients in a pot. Simmer uncovered for 20 minutes, stirring occasionally. Using a hand-held mixer, pulse apples (in the pot), until desired consistency. Add additional cinnamon & xylitol sweetener to personal taste. Add additional water (as needed) to thin, or continue cooking until thicker. The choice is yours. Serve warm or cold.

We love Granny, and her apples.

A.W.E. – *ADD a few raspberries to change the taste and color*
OR – leave apples chunky (more like a compote),
OR – puree completely for a smooth texture

FACT: *Granny smith apples are picked before turning*
red-blush in color, making them lower in sugar.
Apples ripen six to ten times faster at room temperature,
than they do in the refrigerator.

GRANNY'S CRANNIES
(Chunky Cranberry Sauce)

12 oz. bag fresh cranberries
½ cup water
2 cups xylitol sweetener
1 tsp. lemon juice
½ tsp. orange extract

Wash cranberries well. Place them in a medium size pot, covering with cold water. Bring to a boil over medium high heat, then reduce heat to low. Add xylitol, lemon juice, and extract. *(*option: you may choose to slightly crush the berries at this point).* Simmer half an hour, stirring very occasionally. Adjust xylitol as needed to personal taste. Serve warm or cold. Don't just have them AS a side... use them ON your sides (maybe the Grilled Veggies on pg. 138).

*We love Granny,
and her cranberries, too !*

A.W.E. – *ADD orange OR lemon zest*

FACT: *It's true, that a good, ripe cranberry will bounce-thus, its other name...bounce berry!*

OH, DOUGH!

2 cups almond flour
¼ cup chickpea flour
½ tsp. baking soda
1 tsp. guar gum (pg. 220)
¼ tsp. sea salt
3 eggs
1 Tbsp. xylitol sweetener
¼ cup grape seed oil
(or butter, or coconut oil)
Parchment paper

In a large bowl sift almond flour, chickpea flour, baking soda, guar gum, and salt. In a separate bowl whisk eggs, xylitol, and oil. Combine wet ingredients into dry ingredients. Once mixed, allow dough to rest for five minutes. *Dough will be moist and sticky.* Split dough into two portions. Roll dough portions, one at a time, thinly between two pieces of parchment to make two crusts. Grease your baking dishes with coconut oil. Dough breaks easily, so simply fill in any holes as you go. Refrigerate crusts if you are making pies. *note: If using this recipe to make a pie, the filling must be cooked first, as the dough, when baked at 350 degrees, will brown quickly after 20 minutes.*

Whoa...Dough !!

A.W.E. – *ADD cinnamon, additional xylitol and vanilla*
OR – your favorite chopped nuts
OR – 2 Tbsps. unsweetened cocoa powder, 4 Tbsps. xylitol,
and up the butter to ½ cup

FACT: *Sea salt (also known as Bay or Solar salt),*
is typically made by the evaporation of sea water.
It's generally more expensive than table salt,
and contains negligible amounts of iodine.

TOASTED PECAN CRUST

8 Tbsps. butter, softened
1-½ cups pecans, finely chopped
1-¼ cups almond flour
¼ cup chickpea flour
½ cup xylitol sweetener
1 tsp. vanilla extract
pinch of salt
1 tsp. guar gum (pg. 220)

Preheat oven to 325 degrees

Grease (with coconut oil), a large glass pie dish or glass 9 "x13" baking dish. In a bowl, place all ingredients and combine well. Press nut mixture firmly and evenly across the bottom of the baking dish. Bake for 20 minutes. Remove from oven. Crust is ready to use for your choice of fillings for dessert. Gently ladle in your choice of filling, to avoid lifting the crust.

It's all about the nut.

A.W.E. – *use any of your favorite nuts in a crust*

FACT: *There are 1,000 varieties of pecans.*
Pecans should remain fresh in an airtight container in the
refrigerator for about 9 months,
or in the freezer for up to 2 years.

More Helpful Hints and Ideas

- **GLUTEN-FREE BREADCRUMBS:** To make medium-size PORK RIND breadcrumbs, place them in a large zip-top plastic bag, and crush them using a rolling pin. Don't "hammer" them, or you will puncture the bag. To make fine breadcrumbs, use a tabletop blender to grind up the rinds in small batches (so you don't bind your motor). Season them appropriately for recipe selection, or to your personal taste. Try italian seasonings, such as oregano, basil, thyme, and parsley for our Chicken Parm (pg. 159).

- **HERB SPRINKLES**: Keep airtight containers of your favorite herb combo's, to help ease recipe preparation. Combos like: sea salt, parsley, basil, oregano, thyme, paprika, black pepper, marjoram, cayenne, curry powder, celery seed, garlic powder, *OR* - rosemary; italian parsley; fresh basil; garlic powder, oregano, crushed red pepper, sea salt, and black pepper. *These should keep well for about six months.*

- **COCONUT OIL:** is considered to be one of the healthiest dietary oils you can use. It is one of the best sources of medium, and short chain fatty acids, making it a powerhouse food.

- **THE JUICE OF A LEMON:** The acid of a lemon helps dissolve tarnish. A halved lemon dipped in salt or baking powder may be used to brighten copper cookware. When mixed with baking SODA- it will remove stains from plastic food storage containers.

- **CHECK YOUR OVEN** for accuracy every few months. If the temperature is off by more than 15 degrees, it may affect cooking times.

- **CHEESECLOTH** (a natural white cotton cloth) is a kitchen must-have. It comes in fine or coarse varieties, and is lint-free. Cheesecloth is great for squeezing citrus (and avoiding seeds), straining soups or stews, and even bundling herbs for simmering in recipes, to name only a few uses.

- **PEEL GARLIC the EASY WAY** – by placing loose garlic cloves in a zip-top plastic bag and using the flat side of a meat mallet.

BEVERAGES

- **Water, Water, Everywhere**
  - **Coconut Water**
    - **Milk**
    - **Milkshakes**
    - **Hot Cocoa**
  - **Chocolate Milk**
  - **Slushierrrrs**
  - **Smoothierrrrs**
    - **Eggnog**
    - **Coffee**
    - **Tea**
    - **Soda**
  - **Hail to Kale**

Drinking It All In
It's Not Only Water

"In order to change,
we must be sick and tired,
of being sick and tired."

Author Unknown

WATER, WATER, EVERYWHERE

Filtered water (with a high quality filter)
chilled or room temperature

*A normal, healthy adult should drink
ONE OUNCE of water
for every TWO POUNDS of body weight.
If you weigh 150 lbs. you should drink-
75 oz. of water PER DAY.
This does not take into account, illness, sweating, or exertion,
when loss of water increases.*

Hard for you to drink water?

TRY:

* A slice of cucumber in your ice water. It's extremely refreshing.

* Cucumber, water, ice, basil, lime juice, and a pinch of salt in the blender.

* Your favorite crushed berries, and some sweetener of choice,
for a burst of flavor.

* For a sweet change, add your favorite liquid stevia flavor.

* Make a Slushier*rrr* (pg. 35)

* *Berry-Ade:*
3 cups strawberries, 1 cup xylitol sweetener, mashed, allow sit 30 minutes.
Add to blender and puree. Strain. Discard solids. Add 4 cups cold water, and
juice from 4 limes. Chill.

JUST DRINK IT!

A.W.E. – *they're ALL A.W.E.S*

FACT: *70 % of your body is water.
By the time you "feel" thirsty, your body has lost approximately 1% of its water.*

COCONUT WATER

Coconut water is rich in essential electrolytes.
It is also rich in vitamins C & B, magnesium, sodium, and calcium.
Coconut water contains a large amount of protein and dietary fiber.

Plain, chilled, or room temperature...
it's always good!

Flavor it.

Use your favorite berry
(such as raspberry and lime, or raspberry and mint)
with your favorite sweetener,
or favorite flavored liquid stevia extract.

Try using coconut water in your Slushier*rrr*s (pg. 35)
instead of water.

A taste of the tropics.

A.W.E. – *they're ALL A.W.E.S.*

FACT: *Coconut water is an anti-carcinogenic, anti-bacterial,
anti-microbial, and anti-viral food.
Coconut water is the clear liquid inside a fresh coconut,
and unless its shell has been damaged,
is more than likely to be sterile.*

MILK

Plain.
Cold.
Hot.
Flavored.

Raw Organic Whole Milk should be your first choice

Just say moooooo!

A.W.E. *– see ideas for Chocolate Milk (pg. 34)*
OR – for berry flavored milk, see Raspberry Glaze (pg. 216)
Puree recipe before chilling.
Add 1 teaspoon at a time into milk until desired flavor is achieved.
This will work great for ANY berry.

FACT: *Whole milk is a good source of vitamins D & K,*
both of which promote healthy bone growth.

MILKSHAKES

*this recipe requires the use of homemade
xylitol-sweetened ice cream

2 cups ice cream (of your flavor choice)
1 cup whole milk

Everything goes in the blender (or food processor, or in a cup using a wand mixer). For a thicker shake, add ¼ cup milk at a time, until desired consistency. For a thinner shake...add more milk (above the 1 cup), ¼ cup at a time, until desired consistency.

Moo squared.

A.W.E. *– peanut butter & jelly milkshake*
1 cup milk, 3 Tbsps. nut butter, 2 Tbsps. fruit only sweetened berry jelly

FACT: *Whole milk is a good source of B-12, (which promotes cardiovascular health,*
and vitamin A (which supports the immune system).

HOT COCOA

½ cup whole milk
½ cup heavy cream
2 Tbsps. xylitol sweetener
1 Tbsp. cocoa powder, unsweetened
pinch of salt
½ tsp. vanilla extract

Place all ingredients in a saucepan, over medium-high heat and whisk occasionally. Heat through, but do not boil.

Don't wait for winter.

A.W.E. – *lower vanilla extract to ¼ tsp., and ADD ¼ tsp. orange extract*
OR – lower vanilla extract to ¼ tsp., and ADD ¼ tsp. peppermint extract
OR – ADD 6 oz. raspberry puree (strained)

FACT: *Cocoa powder is a good source of protein, potassium, and zinc.*

CHOCOLATE MILK

Option 1:
Chill the Hot Cocoa recipe (above), storing it in a shaker style container.

Option 2:
Use 1 Tbsp. of Orange Chocolate Drizzle (pg. 217) to 8 oz. milk
(more or less to personal taste).

Omit the orange extract, and bump up the vanilla extract. This sauce remains pourable. Keep in airtight container in fridge. *This method does leave a grainier chocolate residue in the bottom of the glass, rather than the chilled Hot Cocoa recipe (above), which only requires mixing.*

Don't wait at all !

A.W.E. – *replace vanilla extract with your favorite flavored extract*

FACT: *Cocoa powder is a very good source of magnesium, fiber, phosphorus, manganese, and copper.*

SLUSHIERrrrS

*this recipe requires a blender

12 ice cubes
4 oz. water, filtered
A handful of fresh berries of your choice,
OR- 2 Tbsps. berry jelly (fruit sweetened only)
sweetener of your choosing

Pour ice cubes into blender and crush. Add water, berries (or jelly), and sweetener of your choice, as necessary. Continue blending until desired consistency *(chunky or pureed).*

Watch out for brain freeze.

A.W.E. – a different recipe:
2 cups lemon juice
1-½ cups each raspberries & blueberries
1 cup xylitol dissolved in 1 cup water
2 additional cups water
Pour into a freezer-proof container, and freeze 8 hours.
Allow to stand 45 minutes before slushy-ing!
Don't drink it all at once.
OR – pour your slushierrrr mixture
into ice cube trays, and then use the
frozen cubes to add a little treat to other drinks

FACT: *In general, BERRIES are naturally high in anti-oxidants, the good compounds that help your body fight disease.*

SMOOTHIERrrrS

1 cup greek yogurt, full-fat
2 cups fresh berries
sweetener of choice
ice cubes as desired for thickness

Everything in the blender! Adjust your sweetener of choice, and the number of ice cubes used, based on how thick you want your smoothierrrr.

OR
1-¼ cups milk
¼ cup cocoa powder, unsweetened
¼ tsp. vanilla extract
pinch of salt
2 Tbsps. xylitol sweetener
¼ cup nut butter
ice cubes as desired for thickness

Everything in the blender, and adjust sweetener, chocolate, vanilla, and nut butter of your choice, to your liking. Love what you eat.

Good 'n smoother.

A.W.E. – *don't be afraid to try flavored liquid stevia extracts,*
OR – *replace yogurt with heavy cream*

FACT: *The darker the color of your berry,*
the higher it is in phytochemical content
(the things that help you fight disease).

EGGNOG

8 egg yolks
¾ cup xylitol sweetener
3 cups whole milk
3 cups heavy cream
4 whole cloves
¼ tsp. ground cinnamon
2 tsps. vanilla extract
⅛ tsp. freshly grated nutmeg

note: recipe requires wire-mesh strainer (or equivalent)

optional garnishes: Whipped Cream (pg. 212), ground cinnamon,
or freshly ground nutmeg

In a large bowl, beat egg yolks until pale and thick. Gradually add xylitol until well blended. In a saucepan over medium heat, heat milk, cloves, and cinnamon, stirring constantly for 8 to 10 minutes (or until bubbles appear at edge of pan). Do not boil. Remove from heat, and pour half of the hot milk mixture into the egg mixture to temper. Return egg mixture back into remaining sauce in pan, and return to heat. Stir constantly for another 6 or 7 minutes, or until mixture coats the back of a spoon evenly (it does this at about 160 degrees). Do not boil. Remove from heat, and add heavy cream. Strain nog through a wire mesh. Allow to cool one hour. Add vanilla and nutmeg. Chill completely. Garnish as desired.

DON'T wait for the holidays!

A.W.E. – *drop vanilla extract to 1 tsp.*
and ADD 1 tsp. peppermint OR almond extract

FACT: *Cloves are known for their numbing effect on mouth tissues.*
They have been used by many doctors in the treatment of digestive,
as well as dental issues for many centuries.

COFFEE

When possible, opt for water-decaffeinated varieties of coffee
to avoid chemical toxicity.
Yes, coffee is typically chemically-decaffeinated.

Drink decaf. Caffeine is not your friend.
*It stimulates the centers of your brain that cause your
sympathetic nervous system to become more active
(the fight or flight response center),
with the end result being a rise in blood sugar.*

Don't forget your hot pot of coffee
may be converted into a batch of your favorite ICED COFFEE.
Plain, or flavored, sweetened, or creamed,
allow your coffee to cool,
and store in the refrigerator until you add ice.

If you make your own coffee, you can make your own hot or chilled Mocha's!
Just add a little unsweetened cocoa powder, the sweetener of your choice, and a
splash of heavy cream, or milk (steamed, or not).

Cuppajoe.

A.W.E. – *try adding these to your coffee filters before brewing:
extracts such as almond; mint; pumpkin; blueberry;
raspberry; hazelnut; or vanilla (or your favorite),
or a dash of nutmeg, cinnamon, or sea salt
(salt helps remove bitterness)*

FACT: *Coffee, even the weak, healthier water-decaffeinated
Varieties, are dehydrating.
For every ounce of weak coffee you consume,
you should consume the equivalent amount in filtered water,
just to keep your insides happy.*

TEA

Make it hot. Drink it cold.

Drink decaf. Caffeine is not your friend.
It stimulates the centers of your brain that cause your
sympathetic nervous system to become more active
(the fight or flight response center)
with the end result being a rise in blood sugar.

Sweet Tea:
3 cups water
2 family-size decaf tea bags
¾ cup xylitol sweetener
7 cups chilled water
1 gallon container

Bring 3 cups of water to boil in a saucepan, and add tea bags. Boil 1 minute then remove from heat. Cover pan and allow tea to steep for 10 minutes. Do not squeeze tea bags, discard them. Add xylitol, stirring until dissolved. Pour 7 cups chilled water into container, and add tea. Keep refrigerated.

Have your tea, and drink it, too.

A.W.E. – *heat 12 oz. frozen blueberries,*
with ¾ cup xylitol sweetener.
Strain. Pour into 4 cups of hot tea. Chill.
OR – pour 4 cups hot tea over 3 cups of fresh blackberries (mashed),
1 Tbsp. fresh mint leaves, chopped, ⅛ tsp. baking soda,
and 1-¼ cups xylitol sweetener.
Allow to stand for 1 hour.
Strain. Add 2 cups cold water.
Chill.

FACT: *Just like coffee, teas*
(even the weak, healthier, water-decaffeinated varieties)
are dehydrating. For every ounce of weak tea you consume,
you should consume the equivalent amount in filtered water,
just to keep your insides happy.
Always use cold fresh-filtered water to make tea. Don't reuse previously heated water.
Don't squeeze your tea bags before discarding them.
Most teas steep between 3 and 7 minutes.

SODA

SODA JUNKIE?
Here are a few good STEVIA-sweetened sodas you may like:

ZEVIA (www.zevia.com)
and
VIRGIL'S ZERO

Both companies have numerous flavors to choose from.
Try to find them in glass bottles, rather than cans,
to eliminate aluminum influences.

*We're all for a bubbly treat now and then,
but don't forget your water.*

Caution ! May cause burping.

A.W.E. – *Or make your own soda using CLUB SODA.
Mix your favorite crushed berries
(with sweetener of your choice),
in a big glass of club soda.*

*OR – ADD your favorite liquid stevia flavors
1 cup carbonated water or club soda with
10 to 15 drops of your favorite liquid stevia sweetener*

*OR – make Cilantro-Ade by using
1 cup seltzer, ½ cup water, 1 cup lime juice,
½ cup xylitol sweetener, and 1 cup cilantro sprigs.
Bring xylitol and water to boil. Remove from heat.
Steep 5 minutes, strain. Chill.
Stir seltzer, lime juice, and 10 Tbsps. chilled xylitol liquid together.*

FACT: *HYDRATION is KEY, to your good health,
but don't count only on soda to do it!*

HAIL TO KALE

2 cups organic kale, washed
½ granny smith apple
8 strawberries
xylitol or stevia sweetener to personal taste
1-½ cups water
juice from ½ lemon

Place all ingredients into a blender or food processor, pulsing until smooth. Served straight-up or over ice…the choice is yours.

Getting a helping of healthy greens...
never tasted this yummy!

Dream green...think drink.

A.W.E. – *LOWER water to ¾ cup, and ADD 6 ice cubes to make*
your kale...slushy
OR – pour it into ice cube trays and freeze
for use in your next glass of water

FACT: *Nutritionally, kale is a powerhouse!*
It contains fiber, calcium, B6, magnesium,
vitamin A, vitamin C, and vitamin K.
It's also a great source for minerals:
copper, potassium, iron, manganese, and phosphorus.

More Helpful Hints and Ideas

- **CHILLIN'**: Make SWEETENED ICE CUBES: raspberry & mint, (or any mashed berry) with a little xylitol sweetener for a surprise.

- **Milk**: In states that permit, buy RAW Organic whole milk, cream, and cheeses, too.

- **SOBE Lifewater**: Their most current flavors are erythritol sweetened, and have no modified food starch in them. Straight off the shelf at the supermarket. At the time of printing, Sobe Lifewater (without sugar) was available in the following flavors: Blood Orange Mango; Acai Raspberry; Kiwi Cherimoya; Yumberry Pomegranate; Fuji Apple Pear; Black and Blue Berry; Black Cherry Dragonfruit, Strawberry Dragonfruit (our kids love the Fuji Apple, Yumberry, and the Black and Blue Berry best –especially as ice pops).

- **Lauric acid** is the main saturated fat in coconut milk (also found in mothers milk), and has been show to promote brain development, and bone health.

- **"DIET DRINKS** are widely promoted to help you lose weight but mounting evidence shows that artificial sweeteners like aspartame cause weight gain rather than weight loss." Dr. Joseph Mercola's article, *Artificial Sweetener May Be Worse than Sugar for Diabetics.*

- **LIME-MINT refresher**: In a small pot add 1 cup water, 1 cup fresh lime juice, 1 cup xylitol sweetener (or stevia equivalent), and ¼ cup of fresh mint leaves torn. Heat over medium heat for 15 minutes. Allow to cool completely. Strain. Pour a little into your club soda or plain seltzer, with ice.

- **Almond-Cherry chiller**: In a small pot add ½ cup water, 1 cup unsweetened cherry juice, ¾ cup xylitol sweetener (or stevia equivalent) over medium heat for 15 minutes. Remove from heat and add 1 tsp. almond extract. Allow to cool completely. Pour a little into your club soda or plain seltzer, with ice.

RISE 'N SHINE

- Coconut "Up-'N-Eat-'Em" Pancakes
  - Wicked-Good Waffles
  - "Mato" 'N Egg Nests
  - Very Berry Muffins
  - Pepper 'N Egg Cradles
  - Mini Scramblers
  - Family-Style Egg Bake
- Nonnie's Bacon 'N Egg Squares
  - Sausage Gravy
  - "Faux" 'Nana Nut Bread
  - Cravin' Coffee Cake

START RIGHT
It Doesn't Have to Be Eggs

"When baking, follow directions.
When cooking, go by your own taste."

Laiko Bahrs
Culinary Consultant

COCONUT "UP-'N-EAT-'EM" PANCAKES

2 eggs
2 Tbsps. heavy cream
1 tsp. xylitol sweetener
2 Tbsps. butter, melted
¼ tsp. vanilla extract
¼ tsp. sea salt
2 Tbsps. coconut flour, sifted
¼ tsp. baking powder
butter or coconut oil (for cooking)

optional: serve with any combination of the following:
Whipped Cream (pg. 212)
fresh berries
Berry Glaze (pg. 216)

In a bowl mix eggs, melted butter, heavy cream, vanilla, xylitol, and salt. In a separate bowl sift coconut flour & baking powder. Combine dry and wet ingredients. Heat the additional Tbsp. of coconut oil or butter in a skillet over medium high heat. Spoon batter onto hot skillet making pancakes 3" in diameter. Cook until lightly browned, and then flip. Top with whipped cream, fresh berries, or berry glaze, as desired. *This recipe yields 8 small pancakes.*

Butter melters.

A.W.E. – *throw some fresh blueberries in the batter.*
These pancakes may be refrigerated and eaten cold or reheated.
The kids will love them as snacks.

FACT: *Baking Powder is still expected to be good, 6 months after opening.*
To test the quality of your baking powder, place a pinch of it in hot water.
If it bubbles, it's still good.
(To test the quality of Baking Soda, place a pinch of it in vinegar.
If it bubbles, it's still good.)

WICKED-GOOD WAFFLES

*note: use of a regular (not Belgian) waffle maker is required

2 cups almond flour
1 tsp. guar gum (pg. 220)
2 tsps. baking powder
6 eggs
½ tsp. vanilla extract
2 Tbsps. xylitol sweetener
½ cup heavy cream (or half & half)
¼ cup club soda
grape seed oil

In a bowl SIFT: almond flour, guar gum, and baking powder. In a second bowl mix eggs, vanilla, xylitol, and heavy cream - whisking well. Plug in waffle maker, allowing it to come to temperature. Combine wet ingredients into dry. Once mixed, add club soda. Using a pastry brush, coat waffle maker lightly with grape seed oil. Pour ¼ cup + 2 Tbsps. of batter in each waffle area. Close waffle iron and cook until desired doneness. Yields 8 to 9 (3" x 4") waffles.

ALWAYS double this recipe. These will be a hit!

Stack 'em high.

A.W.E. – *OMIT vanilla and xylitol and
ADD your favorite herbs and/or cheese,
and use it as an edible "sponge," under a "saucy" entree*

FACT: *National Waffle Day is August 24ᵗʰ.
It is believed that waffles have descended from the flat cakes of ancient Greece.
The Pilgrims are to thank, for bringing waffle irons to the U.S.
If you make too many waffles, you can successfully freeze them,
reheating them in your toaster.*

"MATO" 'N EGG NESTS

4 medium size tomatoes
4 eggs
sea salt and freshly ground black pepper
½ cup mozzarella cheese, shredded
garnish option: shredded fresh basil

Preheat oven to 425 degrees

Slice off the top third of each tomato, and set aside. Scoop out the seeds from each. Place scooped out tomatoes in an 8" x 8" glass baking dish. Crack one egg into each tomato nest. Season with salt and pepper to taste. Replace the cut-off tops of tomato, and bake 10 minutes. Remove the tops, sprinkle mozzarella cheese on top. Cook an additional 5 to 10 minutes, or until cheese is bubbling. Garnish with chopped basil. Serve immediately.

The best nest! Featherless, of course.

A.W.E. *– garnish with cooked, crumbled bacon, and a little oregano*
OR – ADD slices of cubed avocado
OR – place a spoonful of pesto under the egg inside of the tomato
OR – OMIT cheese, and ADD thyme and garlic

FACT: *Tomatoes are the world's most popular fruit.*
They are high in fiber, and rich in vitamins A & C.
Don't store tomatoes in the refrigerator.
Cold temperatures lessen the flavor of tomatoes.

VERY BERRY MUFFINS

Dry ingredients:
3 cups almond flour
½ tsp. sea salt
1-½ tsps. guar gum (pg. 220)
1 cup xylitol sweetener
6 Tbsps. coconut flour
1 tsp. baking powder
¾ cup walnuts, coarsely chopped
¾ pint fresh blueberries

Wet ingredients:
¼ cup coconut oil, melted
1 egg yolk, room temperature
3 eggs, room temperature
1 Tbsp. vanilla extract
note: if eggs are cold, coconut oil will solidify when combining.

11 cupcake liners (we like higher, fuller muffins)
2 tsps. xylitol sweetener, finely ground
(in a coffee bean grinder)

Preheat oven to 350 degrees

Mix all dry ingredients (except for blueberries). In a separate bowl mix all wet ingredients. Once combined, stir wet ingredients into dry ingredients. Batter will become very thick (it may be too thick for your mixer). Incorporate blueberries. Place liners in muffin pan. Add a heaping Tbsp. of batter in each liner. Before adding more batter, push down on existing batter to fill air voids. Scoop remaining batter and distribute equally among the 11 liners. *This batter does not rise.* Muffins will come out of the oven looking *exactly* how they did going into the oven. Bake 30 minutes (about 20 minutes for mini's), or until tops are lightly browned, and a toothpick comes out clean. Remove and sprinkle a pinch of powdered xylitol over the top of each muffin while hot. These will be a hit, cold or hot! Keep refrigerated. *These muffins freeze well in zip-top freezer bags for future use.*

Who needs a bakery.

A.W.E. – *substitute strawberries for blueberries*

FACT: *Blueberries have significant anti-bacterial,
and anti-viral compounds.
They are the second most popular berry consumed in the U.S.,
strawberries being the first.*

The Newest DIRTY DOZEN
*The HIGHEST pesticide contamination resides in these fruits & veggies.
ALWAYS buy organic! The twelve MOST contaminated are:*

Apples
Carrots *
Celery
Cherries
Grapes *
Kale
Lettuce
Nectarines *
Peaches *
Pears *
Strawberries
Sweet Bell Peppers

**A low-glycemic eating plan would NOT include
these fruits or veggies*

PEPPER 'N EGG CRADLES

1 Tbsp. coconut oil
1 large bell pepper (any color), cut into four ½" thick rings
4 large eggs
sea salt and freshly ground black pepper

Cut off top and bottom of the pepper, and make 4 even-size ½" strips (across the width of the pepper). Make sure cuts are straight so that pepper slices sit flat in a pan. Remove seeds, and ribs, leaving rings of pepper, whole. In a large skillet, heat oil over medium-high heat. Add pepper rings to pan, and cook 3 minutes. Flip pepper rings and allow to cook 2 minutes. Then crack one egg into the middle of each of the pepper cradles. Season with salt and pepper. Cook until the egg whites are mostly set, but yolks still runny. *This should take 2 to 3 minutes. (If you made a side of bacon, cook the peppers in bacon fat, and spoon three tsps. of bacon fat on top of yolk to help it set before flipping.)* Flip pepper cradles. Cook 1 additional minute, or until desired yolk firmness. Serve hot.

Pepper, pepper, bo-bepper.

A.W.E. – *top cooked eggs with chunky salsa*
OR – *use red, or yellow bell peppers, rather than green*
OR – *sprinkle the tops of the eggs with crumbled, cooked sausage,*
and cooked, chopped onion before flipping

FACT: *Green bell peppers are slightly less sweet*
than yellow or orange peppers, and a little more bitter.
A red bell pepper, is merely a ripened green bell pepper.

MINI SCRAMBLERS

8 eggs
½ cup milk
½ cup turkey, cooked, crumbled
(or sausage, ham, or bacon)
⅓ cup swiss cheese
(or mozzarella, or cheddar)
sea salt and freshly ground black pepper
24 cup mini cupcake baking tin
24 paper liners

Preheat oven to 375 degrees

Place paper liners in your muffin tin. In a large bowl whisk eggs and milk. Add turkey, most of the cheese, and salt & pepper. Mix well and ladle egg mixture into liners. Sprinkle remaining cheese on top. Bake minis for 8 to 10 minutes. Serve hot. Refrigerate leftovers.

Your kids will love these! Make their favorite combo's. They're great cold, which makes them easy to grab-n'-go. If you add any veggies, remember to sauté them first. This eliminates extra water they would otherwise add to your eggs. There's nothing worse than a wet mini.

Now, scram!

A.W.E. – *ADD chopped, cooked spinach and sautéed onions*
OR – OMIT milk and add heavy cream or ½ & ½

FACT: *Rather than stirring your eggs with a spoon,*
push them with a spatula to make them fluffier.
When adding cheese to your eggs, cubed cheeses will leave gooey
pockets to come across, where shredded cheese will dissolve.

FAMILY-STYLE EGG BAKE

10 eggs
1 cup milk (or heavy cream)
3 Tbsps. almond flour
2 Tbsps. coconut flour
1 Tbsp. dijon mustard
3 cups cheddar cheese, shredded
sea salt and freshly ground black pepper
2 pkgs. frozen spinach, thawed, drained, chopped

Preheat oven to 350 degrees

In a bowl whisk milk, almond flour, and coconut flour. Add eggs, mustard, salt and pepper. Pour into greased (with coconut oil) 10" x 15" glass baking dish. Add 1-½ cups of the cheese to egg mixture, and then evenly layer spinach over the top. Bake 10 to 12 minutes until the edges of your baked omelet are set, and then sprinkle with remaining cheddar cheese, baking 5 more minutes or until cheese is melted. Remove from oven. Slice and serve.

Pass the baking dish.
Real men eat egg-bake.

A.W.E. – *ADD sliced ham or prosciutto*
OR – ADD any of your favorite omelet ingredients
OR – ADD a dash of tabasco, hot sauce, salsa, or cajun spices
and serve with sour cream

FACT: *To keep your eggs from*
becoming overly "wet and watery," ALWAYS pre-cook your veggies.

NONNIE'S BACON 'N EGG SQUARES

8 slices of thick cut bacon, cut in half
4 eggs
1 Tbsp. dried oregano
sea salt and freshly ground black pepper

Cook bacon (in a large saucepan), three-quarters of the way to desired doneness. Overlap 4 pieces of bacon to make four equal squares in your pan. Crack one egg into the center of each bacon square. Season to taste with salt and pepper. Sprinkle oregano equally on top of the yolks. Allow eggs to cook about 3 minutes. Using a tablespoon, spoon bacon fat over the top of each yolk, until a white film forms, cooking egg from the top down. Cook eggs to your liking.

Bet you can't eat just one.

A.W.E. – *ADD a slice of muenster (or your favorite) cheese to the top*
OR – ADD thinly sliced pieces of avocado on top before adding cheese
OR – serve on top of a medium-thick slice of fresh tomato
OR – serve over a bed of sautéed spinach
OR – serve on top of your favorite hamburger

FACT: *Crack your eggs against a flat surface (like the kitchen counter),*
rather than the edge of a bowl or pan.
This will help you avoid pushing pieces of shell
into your eggs.

SAUSAGE GRAVY

*Biscuits (pg. 6) should be made prior

1 pound ground sausage (no sugar added)
8 slices of thick cut bacon, chopped
½ cup onion, chopped
2 cloves of garlic, minced
1-½ Tbsps. chickpea flour
1-½ Tbsps. almond flour
1 cup heavy cream
1 cup half & half
2 Tbsps. butter
sea salt and freshly ground black pepper

In a pan combine the sausage, bacon, onion, and garlic. Cook on medium-high heat for 10 to 15 minutes, or until sausage is brown and crumbly. Add chickpea and almond flours to pan. Cook 2 minutes, stirring frequently. Add heavy cream and butter, and season with salt and pepper to personal taste. Reduce heat to low, and simmer until thickened. Serve warm over plain biscuits.

Biscuit, or spoon? Hmmmm.

A.W.E. – *ADD ½ cup diced red bell pepper*

FACT: *Chickpea flour is also known
as besan flour and garbanzo bean flour.
While typical flour derives from milled wheat grains
and is often bleached, chickpea flour typically contains nothing
but pure, ground chickpeas.
Chickpea flour has a slightly nutty flavor,
and each serving has significant amounts of iron, phosphorous, and protein.*

"FAUX" 'NANA NUT BREAD

DRY ingredients:
3 cups almond flour
½ tsp. sea salt
1-½ tsps. guar gum (pg. 220)
1 cup + 2 tsps. xylitol sweetener, finely ground
(in a coffee grinder)
6 Tbsps. coconut flour
1 tsp. baking powder
¾ cup walnuts, coarsely chopped

WET ingredients:
¼ cup coconut oil, melted
1 egg yolk, room temperature
3 eggs, room temperature
2 tsps. banana extract

**note: If eggs are cold,
coconut oil will solidify when combining*

Preheat oven to 350 degrees

In a large bowl, mix all DRY ingredients (except for walnuts). In a separate bowl mix all WET ingredients. Combine wet ingredients into dry ingredients. Stir well. Batter will become very thick. Add walnuts. Place batter in an 8"x8" greased (with coconut oil) glass baking dish. Bake 35 to 40 minutes, or until top is lightly browned, and a toothpick comes out clean. **note: this freezes well.*

NaNah lovers...smile.

A.W.E. – *ADD strawberries and/or blueberries*

FACT: *Not only is coconut oil one of the healthiest oils you can consume, but it is one of the best moisturizers for your skin. It's readily absorbed and isn't greasy.*

CRAVIN' COFFEE CAKE

Crumb Topping:
¼ cup granulated coconut nectar
¼ cup Faux Brown Sugar (pg. 23)
2 packets truvia sweetener
¼ cup + 2 Tbsps. almond flour
2 Tbsps. coconut flour
1 tsp. ground cinnamon
½ cup butter, softened
¾ cup pecans, chopped

Batter:
½ cup pecans, medium-coarse chopped
1 cup butter, softened
2-½ cups xylitol sweetener
2 Tbsps. granulated coconut nectar
2 Tbsps. Faux Brown Sugar (pg. 23)
7 eggs
2-½ cups almond flour
½ cup coconut flour
2 tsps. guar gum (pg. 220)
½ tsp. baking soda
8 oz. sour cream
2 tsps. vanilla extract
coconut or grape seed oil (to grease ramekins)

For crumb topping: combine coconut nectar, Faux Brown Sugar, truvia, almond flour, coconut flour, and cinnamon. Once mixed, add butter and blend. Add pecans and set aside. *Preheat oven to 350 degrees.* For cake: Bake your pecans 7 minutes on a parchment-lined cookie sheet. Remove and set aside, allowing to cool 20 minutes. For the batter: In a VERY large mixing bowl, beat butter until creamy, then add xylitol, coconut nectar, Faux Brown Sugar, and eggs (one at a time). In a small bowl SIFT: almond flour, coconut flour, guar gum, and baking soda. Slowly add the dry ingredients and the sour cream (alternating each, and combining well in between each addition) into the butter mixture. Add vanilla. Grease seven 4" ramekins with oil and add ¼ cup + 2 Tbsps. batter to each (flattening to cover bottom of ramekins). Sprinkle each ramekin with enough crumb mixture to cover, and then sprinkle with toasted pecans. On top of the crumb/pecans layer, add another ¼ cup + 2 Tbsps. batter (flattening again). Top each ramekin with remaining crumb mixture, and toasted pecans. Bake 43 to 46 minutes, or until toothpick inserted comes out clean. *note: if you use smaller ramekins, you must drastically reduce cooking time. Store any remaining cakes in an airtight container in the refrigerator. Freeze for up to 2 months.

Milk? Tea? Or coffee side?

A.W.E. – *OMIT vanilla and ADD maple extract*

FACT: *Granulated coconut nectar,*
is made from the flower buds of coconut trees.
Although similar to table sugar on the glycemic index
(use it sparingly), granulated coconut nectar is unrefined.

COFFEE TIDBITS
(we suggest organically grown,
water-decaffeinated brands of coffee)

- All coffee in the word grows in the "bean belt." The area between the Tropics of Cancer and Capricorn.

- Hawaii is the only U.S. state that grows coffee.

- The second-most widely used product in the world, after oil, is coffee.

- A coffee tree may flower up to 8 times a year.

- USED coffee grounds may be added to compost or mulch. Acid-loving plants such as blueberries, love them.

More Helpful Hints and Ideas

- **ALWAYS START WITH LEFTOVERS**: You've already cooked once. Use it to your advantage! Breakfast doesn't HAVE to be eggs.

- **LOOKING for a BOWL of something**: Cereal may be out...but our "Faux" Nola, Homemade Granola (pg. 61), is in! Get a bowl, and add some whole milk.

- **What INGREDIENTS can you use in your Scramblers or Omelets**: Bacon, Tomatoes, Cheeses, Onions (green, white, leek. shallot, chive), Mushrooms, Peppers, Protein, Fresh herbs, Salsa, Veggies...be creative! Cook veggies first, to eliminate excess water.

- **GREEK YOGURT**: Add some fresh berries (whole or mashed) and your favorite sweetener. Top with some "Faux" Nola, Homemade Granola (pg. 61).

- *SMOOTHIERrrrS*: (pg. 36) for breakfast on the go!

- **EAT-YOUR-SPINACH SQUARES** (pg. 88).

- **Leftover meatloaf**: Is awesome reheated with a fried egg on top. **Baked eggs in avocados**: Baked avocados filled with an egg in a 425 degree oven. Cut a little off of bottom of avocado half, so that it sits flat in a greased baking dish, and add an egg with s&p, maybe a crumble of cooked bacon or sausage on top, or cheese and cook about 15 to 20 minutes, or until egg is cooked to desired doneness.

- **See A Tisket A BISCUIT** (pg. 6) for your yolk dipping.

- **PUT YOUR EGGS TO BED**: Serve your favorite style of eggs over a bed of wilted, sautéed spinach OR blanched asparagus. With or without bacon, cheese, or sauce on top.

- **FLAXSEED MUFFINS**: Mix 3 Tbsps. ground flaxseed, 1 Tbsp. almond flour, 1 tsp. cinnamon, 1 tsp. coconut oil (melted), 1 tsp. baking powder, pinch guar gum, pinch salt, 1 tsp. Nature's Hollow xylitol-sweetened honey, pinch stevia sweetener, 1 egg. Place in a ramekin and microwave for 1 minute 15 seconds.

ON-THE-GO

- **"Faux" Nola**
  Homemade Granola
- **"Faux" Nola Bars**
  Homemade Granola Bars
- **Humpty Dumpty Salad**
- **Ham-It-Up Salad**
- **Lovin' Lobster Salad**
- **A & A Chicken Salad**
- **Coconut Shrimp 'N Curry Salad**
- **Cumba-Wich**
- **Garlicky-'Cado Spread**
- **Rolled 'N Ready Ideas**
- **Pass the Kale Chips**
- **Fruit Roll 'Em Ups**
- **Go...Nuts**
- *EATING OUT Suggestions*

LIFE'S A PICNIC
Lunch Doesn't Have to Be Boring

**"Ask not what you can
do for your country.
Ask what's for lunch."**

Orson Welles
American Actor, Writer, Director, Producer
1915 - 1985

"FAUX" NOLA
Homemade Granola (without the grains)

note: read your labels carefully.
Most dehydrated/dried berries have sugar added.
Make your own by soaking them in xylitol-sweetened water,
before dehydrating.

1 cup unsweetened coconut, flaked, toasted
1 cup peanuts, toasted
(If you want a chunkier, easier-to-grab granola, leave nuts whole.
To use it as a topping, chop them smaller.)
1 cup pecans, chopped, toasted
1 cup almonds, sliced, toasted
1 cup dried raspberries (or berry of your choice)
powdered sweetener (type and amount of your choice)

This recipe is great on its own, added to yogurt,
or sprinkled on top of ice cream.

Preheat oven to 350 degrees

Place coconut flakes on a parchment lined baking sheet. Bake 3 to 4 minutes, or until light brown in color. Remove from oven and place in a bowl. While warm, sprinkle on your powdered sweetener and stir well. Place nuts on the parchment lined baking sheet. Bake 7 to 8 minutes. Remove from oven and mix with coconut. Once completely cool, add berries and toss. Store in airtight containers.

Crunchy. Sweet. Crunchy. Sweet.

A.W.E. – *ADD milk to make it a "cereal"*
OR – ADD walnuts or macadamia nuts
OR – ADD broken up pieces of malitol-sweetened chocolate, (pg. 219)

FACT: *Only 5% of cranberries are sold fresh.*
The remaining 95% are turned into cranberry sauce,
cranberry juice, and other cranberry products.

"FAUX" NOLA BARS
Homemade Granola Bars (without the grains)

*note: this recipe requires the making of
"Faux" Nola (pg. 61), prior to preparation.
It is recommended to use a finer chop for nuts when making bars.
Best results achieved with an overnight in refrigerator.

½ cup butter, softened
¼ cup + 2 Tbsps. xylitol sweetener
1 egg yolk
½ tsp. vanilla extract
2 Tbsps. fruit-only sweetened jelly (no sugar added)
Flavor of choice to go with your "Faux" Nola flavor
1 cup almond flour
¼ cup chickpea flour
1 tsp. guar gum (pg. 220)
½ cup unsweetened coconut, shredded
1 to 1-¼ cups "Faux" Nola

Preheat oven to 350 degrees

In a bowl combine butter and xylitol. Add egg, vanilla, and jelly, stirring well. Sift in almond flour, chickpea flour, and guar gum, mix until completely combined. Fold in shredded coconut and "Faux" Nola. Press batter into 7" x 11" greased (with coconut oil) glass baking dish, and bake 22 to 25 minutes, until edges are golden brown, or a toothpick inserted into the center comes out clean. Allow to cool completely. Refrigerate overnight. Cut into bars. Keep refrigerated in snack-size zip-top bags. Grab and go made simple.

Who needs a vending machine?

A.W.E. – *OMIT vanilla extract and ADD berry flavored extract (of choice)*

FACT: *Almond flour is made from almonds without skin that are blanched and ground into flour. It is a low carbohydrate alternative to wheat flour.*

HUMPTY DUMPTY SALAD

12 eggs, hardboiled, peeled, chopped
1 cup Mayonnaise (pg. 7)
3 avocados, peeled, pitted, cubed
4 stalks celery, halved, diced
½ cup vidalia onion, minced
3 Tbsps. dill pickle, diced
2 Tbsps. stone-ground mustard
sea salt & freshly ground black pepper

Place chopped eggs in a bowl and add all ingredients. Season with salt and pepper to personal taste. More mayo, onion, pickle, mustard...you decide! Refrigerate in an airtight container until ready to use.

Get eggy with it.

A.W.E. – *OMIT pickles and ADD capers*
OR – *OMIT pickles and ADD curry powder*

FACT: *One large egg has the same amount of protein*
as in 1 oz. of meat, fish, or poultry.
Most people consume eggs from chickens.
Currently, worldwide, there are well over 200 breeds of chicken.

HAM – IT – UP SALAD

1 lb. cooked ham, julienned
(or coarsely chopped)
½ cup sour pickle, julienned
(or coarsely chopped)
½ cup Mayonnaise (pg. 7)
¾ tsp. mustard
¼ tsp. freshly ground black pepper
(or more to taste)

Place all ingredients in a medium bowl and mix well. Serve on a bed of your favorite greens, on a cucumber hero (Cumba-Wich, pg. 68), or rolled up in a large lettuce leaf. Anyway you make it, it will taste good.

Add the mustard...hold the rye !

A.W.E. – *ADD ½ tsp. prepared horseradish*
OR – ADD 1 to 2 hard-boiled eggs, crumbled

FACT: *Julienning your vegetables, cheeses, or proteins,*
adds visual interest and appeal to your food.

LOVIN' LOBSTER SALAD

1 lb. lobster meat, cooked and chopped
1 lb. shrimp, deveined, cooked and chopped
2 Tbsps. fresh tarragon
2 Tbsps. dijon mustard
½ cup Mayonnaise (pg. 7)
½ cup sour cream
4 celery stalks, thinly sliced
1 green onion, (or leek), sliced
1 red bell pepper, julienned
sea salt and freshly ground black pepper
baby spinach (as a serving bed)
4 eggs, hardboiled, crumbled (as garnish)
lemon, sliced (as garnish)

Place lobster and shrimp in a large bowl. In a small bowl, mix sour cream, mayonnaise, tarragon, mustard, onion, red pepper, celery, salt, and pepper. Mix well. Add sour cream mixture to lobster/shrimp. Once combined, refrigerate until ready to eat. Serve on a bed of baby spinach (or your favorite greens). Garnish with crumbled egg and a slice of lemon.

Lovin' me some lobster.

A.W.E. – *ADD cooked, crumbled bacon*
OR – ADD grape tomato halves
OR – ADD 1 cup cooked green beans, diced
OR – serve in rolled-up lettuce leaves

FACT: *Leeks have a mild, sweet taste and are less bitter than scallions.*
Choose leeks that have a stalk
(the light green color between the white end and the darker top),
that are less than 1-½" in length.
The dark green tops should be strong, not wilted, and without blemish.

A & A CHICKEN SALAD
(Avocado & Apple)

1 cups chicken, cooked, cubed
½ cup granny smith apple, diced
¼ cup celery, chopped
2 Tbsps. pecans, chopped, toasted
¼ cup flat-leaf parsley, chopped
2 Tbsps. red onion, chopped
5 small fresh mint, chopped
¾ tsp. jalapeño pepper
¼ tsp. sea salt
1 Tbsp. lemon juice
½ tsp. olive oil
½ avocado, pitted, peeled, diced

In a medium bowl, combine everything except for the avocado. Mix well. Stir in half of the avocado, mashing it into ingredients. Add remaining diced avocado, and stir lightly. Serve over your favorite greens, piled high on slices of granny smith apples, or on a Cumba-wich (pg. 68).

Ahhhhh-vocado makes it perfect.

A.W.E. – *OMIT jalapeño pepper*
OR – substitute your favorite toasted nuts, for pecans
OR – a new recipe suggestion:
try your chicken salad with pecans, mayonnaise, tarragon, lemon zest,
lemon juice, granny smith apples, celery, and red onion

FACT: *Chicken is a very good source of protein, niacin, and selenium.*
Chicken eggs aren't only white, or shades of brown;
they also come in shades of blue and green.

COCONUT SHRIMP 'N CURRY SALAD

1 lb. shrimp; cleaned, deveined, cooked and chunked
⅓ cup Mayonnaise (pg. 7)
3 Tbsps. shredded coconut, unsweetened
3 Tbsps. sour cream
1-½ tsps. curry powder
1 tsp. lemon juice
2 scallions, minced
freshly ground black pepper to taste
large leaf lettuce of your choice

Mix all ingredients except for lettuce. Refrigerate until cold. Serve on top of, or rolled up in, your lettuce leaves.

HURRY! Curry!

A.W.E. – *OMIT shrimp and ADD cubed chicken*
OR – OMIT onion powder and ADD scallions
and ADD a little finely chopped celery, for extra crunch

FACT: *Watercress and arugula add a "spicy" punch.*
Due to its high iodine content, watercress has a strengthening
effect on the thyroid gland.

CUMBA-WICH

As many cucumbers, as you want sandwiches
Cold cuts, salads, or cheeses of your choice
Garnishes of your choice

Peel cucumbers. Cut cucumbers lengthwise, end-to-end. Run a spoon (or melon-baller) down the center, and remove all seeds, plus some flesh, leaving a hollowed center, running the length of the cucumber. Allow cucumber to rest on top of a paper towel before sandwich preparation.

"WICH" Ideas:

- Turkey, mozzarella cheese, mesclun greens, with pesto
- Roast beef, havarti cheese, tatziki sauce, with roasted peppers
- Chicken, shrimp, tuna, or your favorite homemade salad
- Sliced shrimp topped with No Skimpin' Shrimpin' (Cocktail Sauce) (pg. 10)
- Ham, muenster cheese, green olives, and spicy mustard
- Leftover meatloaf
- Hamburgers, or cheeseburgers, with all of your favorite trimmings, including Mayonnaise (pg. 7) or Ketchup (pg. 8)

Cuke cute.

A.W.E. – *cut cucumber into slices (width-wise),
and spoon some of your favorite salads
in-between two slices, for bite-size, crunchy, mini-wiches*

FACT: *Having an enclosed seed, and developing from a flower,
in the botanical world, cucumbers are actually fruits.
They contain over 90% water.*

GARLICKY-'CADO SPREAD

1 avocado, halved, peeled, diced
⅓ cup greek yogurt, plain
2 tsps. fresh garlic cloves, minced
1 tsp. lemon juice
1 tbsp. fresh basil leaves, chopped
½ tsp. sea salt
freshly ground black pepper to taste

Put all ingredients in a blender (or food processor), and pulse until smooth. Store refrigerated in an airtight container. Your roll-ups never tasted so good!

Let's wrap!

A.W.E. – *OMIT lemon and ADD lime*
AND/OR – *OMIT basil and ADD cilantro*

FACT: *Garlic keeps longer if the tops remain in place.*
Typically, garlic is hung or braided
(in strands called plaits or gappes),
and stored in a warm & dry place to help it remain dormant.

ROLLED 'N READY IDEAS

Leave them rolled or cut them into 1" pieces,
and hold them together with a toothpick (don't eat the wood).

Romaine wrapped on the outside or cold cuts on the outside-
it doesn't matter how you roll!

- Turkey, cream cheese, sliced cucumber, avocado
- Turkey, havarti cheese, Mayonnaise (pg. 7), fresh dill
- Turkey, brie, fresh rosemary, with mesclun on the inside, and a little oil and vinegar
- Turkey, cream cheese, Cranberry Sauce (pg. 25)
- Turkey, muenster roasted peppers, Mayonnaise (pg. 7), with baby spinach on the inside
- Ham, muenster, grape tomatoes, grape tomatoes
- Roast beef, swiss cheese, cucumber, horseradish Mayonnaise (pg. 7), with baby spinach on the inside
- Roast beef, sliced cheddar, "Matoey" BBQ Sauce (pg. 20), bacon
- Roast beef, horseradish Mayonnaise (pg. 7), swiss cheese, with a sour pickle spear in the middle
- Tuna, chicken (pg. 66), turkey, ham (pg. 64), lobster (pg. 65), egg (pg. 63), or shrimp salad 'with sliced sour pickles for crunch, wrapped in romaine
- Roasted red peppers, fresh basil, fresh mozzarella cheese, with a little balsamic vinegar
- Grilled Veggies (pg. 138), with Balsamic Vinaigrette (pg. 123) in romaine lettuce
- B.L.T.- Strips of bacon, fresh sliced tomatoes, and Mayonnaise (pg. 7) wrapped in romaine (add turkey)

Rollin' with the lunches.

FACT: *The body uses protein to:*
* Renew and/or repair cells & tissue * Make body proteins such as enzymes, some hormones & antibodies * Supply us with energy

Pass the KALE CHIPS

1 bunch of organic kale
1 Tbsp. grape seed, or non-hydrogenated peanut oil
sea salt

Preheat oven to 400 degrees

Wash and dry kale. Tear leaves off of the thick stems, and tear into bite-size pieces. Cover kale with oil and salt. Place kale on parchment lined baking sheet. Bake 15 minutes, or until edges are brown. Kale should be crispy to the touch.

Inhale the kale.

A.W.E. – *toss with parmesan, or asiago cheese,
and your favorite seasonings
OR – ADD 1 Tbsp. creole seasoning or cayenne pepper
OR – cook 3 pieces of bacon until crisp.
Remove from oil, crumble and set aside.
Toss bacon drippings with 1 bunch of torn kale.
Place on parchment-lined, rimmed baking sheet.
Bake at 400 degrees for 10 to 15 minutes.
Toss with bacon crumbles.*

FACT: *Always buy organic kale.
Kale is very high in beta carotene, vitamins K & C, and lutein.*

FRUIT ROLL 'EM UPS

*note: this recipe requires extended cooking time.

1 lb. fresh strawberries
½ cup xylitol sweetener
1-½ tsps. lemon juice
1 piece parchment paper
(wide and long enough to completely cover baking sheet)
1 baking sheet (with a lip)

Preheat oven to 170 degrees

Wash berries and remove stems. Cut into quarters, and place in blender. Add xylitol, and lemon juice. Puree all ingredients, until you have a fine pulp. Line the lipped baking sheet completely with a solid piece of parchment paper, but make sure to leave a few inches overhang on each side (to "tuck" the ends under the sheet while baking, preventing the parchment from falling on top of the fruit while baking/drying.). Fold the parchment well in the corners, so that it lies flat in the baking sheet. Bake for approximately 8 hours, turning the baking sheet every two hours. When done, turn oven off, but allow fruit to stay on the rack. Remove from oven once completely cooled. Using a sharp knife, cut fruit into strips, leaving the parchment on. Roll and store fruit rolls in an airtight container. *DO NOT refrigerate. They will not be pliable, and will rip or break.*

Whether...to leather?

A.W.E. – *SUBSTITUTE any berry for strawberry.*
You can strain seeds of any fruit used (if desired)

FACT: *Strawberry plants may be grown INDOORS,*
but require as much sun as possible. Water your strawberry plants
in the morning to avoid common leaf diseases.

Go...NUTS
(Spicy Pecans)

Spicy Pecans:
2 cups pecan halves
¼ cup xylitol sweetener
1 tsp. water
1 egg white
½ tsp. allspice
1 tsp. cinnamon
⅛ tsp. freshly ground black pepper

Preheat oven to 250 degrees

Whisk egg white, and water in small bowl until frothy. Add pecans, xylitol, cinnamon, allspice, and pepper. Mix well. Place nuts in a single layer, inside a large glass baking dish (greased with coconut oil). Bake for 30 minutes, stir once, making sure to leave nuts in a single layer. Cook an additional 30 minutes or until dry. Cool completely. Store in airtight containers.

Don't GO hungry. GO nuts !

A.W.E. – *Although a great anytime snack,
try using them as a spicy crouton in salads
OR – spice up your favorite nut combo with
cayenne, rosemary, salt, and a little sweetener*

FACT: *Nuts have been an integral part of the
human diet since the beginning of time.*

EATING OUT
Suggestions for eating in the real world

Some words of encouragement. When choosing to eat for health and wellness, people's perceptions do come into play for most of us. You and you alone, are responsible for the choices you make in a public environment. These choices will directly affect how your body heals, or maintains health. You should not be "concerned" with what other people think. This can be difficult for many people, who spend time trying to "fit in" with others. Ultimately, the choices are *yours*. Don't give into peer pressure. Make the right choices for your health. *You're worth it!*

BURGER PLACES:

Triple burgers with cheese, skip the ketchup, have the mayo and mustard, onions, pickles, tomatoes and NO bun. Skip the fries. Still hungry? Sandwiches without bread. Have a second, or perhaps, a side salad, and bottled water.

CHINESE:

Skip all rice (even brown), noodles, anything battered, fortune cookies, and all sweetened sauces. Many asian dishes contain corn starch as a thickener, which should be avoided. Wheat-free varieties of soy sauce (made outside of the U.S., to avoid GMO exposure), are soy products considered safe to eat, due to fermentation. Stick with steamed proteins and veggies. Bottled water.

GREEK:

Grilled meats and proteins (including fish), villager or greek salads. Skip rice and pasta. Bottled water.

MEXICAN:

Order fajitas, enchiladas, soft tacos, or hard tacos...with the fixings (guacamole, sour cream, or pico de gallo), but skip eating the shells. Chili Relleno is a good option (cooked green pepper with ground beef or cheese), make sure they don't use rice as a filler.

TRADITIONAL RESTAURANTS:

Pass on the bread and breadsticks. Make wise decisions on your appetizers (maybe tomato & mozzarella salad, cheese plate, or shrimp cocktail without cocktail sauce (but a sprinkle of lemon), or a cold antipasto salad), soups (are hard to do without knowing what's in them), and salads use oil & vinegar to avoid sugar or toxin exposures. Ask that your entrée be served without rice, pasta, or potato, and have them substituted with additional vegetables (no peas, carrots, or corn) with butter. Dessert, fresh berries (with a side of heavy cream). Bottled water.

ITALIAN:

Order caprese salad (fresh tomato & mozzarella cheese), or a cold antipasto dish. Consider a specialty salad (with nuts, meats, cheese, and oil & vinegar or lemon juice). Order grilled or oven-roasted proteins, with sautéed sides of broccoli rabé, escarole, spinach, etc. Skip the pasta.

Pizza? Easy. Order 4 to 8 slices of your favorite pizza. Ask for a plate, knife and a fork. Scrap off all of the toppings and pile it high...then throw out the crust (no, this isn't sacrilegious), or politely give the serving tray back (you could even order a stuffed calzone, and eat the middle only). A side salad, and you fit right in. Almost. Bottled water.

JAPANESE:

Sashimi. Or, order sushi without rice. Many places will accommodate you by making your sushi with cucumber or seaweed only, when omitting rice. Order a seaweed salad, or hibachi meats and proteins. Don't order anything "spicy" (such as spicy tuna), which have "sirachi" (which has sugar). Use extra wasabi if you like heat.

More Helpful Hints and Ideas

- **What can you put in your ROLL-UPS?**: Mayonnaise (pg. 7), sour pickles, tomatoes, bacon, cheese, cucumber slices, peppers, onions, cream cheese, olives, artichokes, or any spread, dip or veggie you like.

- **Lettuce doesn't have to be on the outside**: Your meat or cheese can be, and your lettuce can be whole, or shredded on the inside! See more ideas at Party Pleasin' Pinwheels (pg. 95).

- **Cut your Grannies**: Make slices of Granny Smith Apples and take them in an airtight container with water and a splash of lemon juice. They won't brown and will stay crunchy.

- **Sliced Apple**: With any nut butter of your choosing *(without sugar of course)*, or cheese slices (like sharp cheddar).

- **Greek Style Yogurt**: Full-fat (of course), with fresh berries, fruit-only sweetened jelly, and/or sweetener of your choice. Why not top it with "Faux" Nola (Homemade Granola (pg. 61).

- **Of course there's always a salad idea**: or two, starting on pg. 111.

- **Yogurt Dip:** Mix 6 oz. Greek yogurt, ⅓ cup nut butter- dip apples or strawberries.

- **Don't let ANY restaurant intimidate you**. There is always something you can have guilt-free. Sometimes it just takes a little ingenuity, and some special requests to get it done.

- **Make your bacon the bread**: BLT's the easy way. For two sandwiches, take 12 pieces of bacon (starting with 6 pieces side by side on your parchment lined baking sheet), and weave them in an over/under pattern. Bake 35 – 40 minutes in a 400 degree oven. Cut into bread shape pieces and allow to cool. Top with lettuce, tomato, salt & pepper and your favorite flavored or plain mayonnaise.

APPETIZERS

- Devilish Eggs
- No-Bones Buffalo Chicken Dip
- Pete's Smokin' Fish Spread
- Sausage 'N Pepper Pie
- Bubblin' Crab Dip
- Chill-E Crab Dip
- Holy Guacamole!
- Let Your Piggy Roll
- Baked Brie
- Eat-Your-Spinach Squares
- Jalapeño Cheese 'Ems
- Stuffed "Matoes"
- "Faux" Sushi
- "Cool-As-A-Cucumba" Dip
- Strawberry Salsa
- Clams Casino
- Party Pleasin' Pinwheels

Awesome Appetizers
Entertain in Good Health

**"To keep the body in
good health is a duty...
otherwise we shall not be able to
keep our mind strong and clear."**

Buddha
Enlightened Being
2500 years ago, India

DEVILISH EGGS

12 hard-boiled eggs
¾ cup Mayonnaise (pg. 7)
1 tsp. spicy brown mustard
⅛ tsp. celery salt
⅛ tsp. sea salt
⅛ tsp. freshly ground black pepper
*(white pepper may be substituted,
so that you do not see "flecks" in the egg yolk mixture)*

*garnish option: Paprika – OR a piece of cooked bacon
OR – a piece of sliced green manzanilla olive.*

After hard-boiling eggs (see FACT below), remove shells and slice lengthwise (end-to-end). Remove yolks and mash in a mixing bowl until crumbly. Place egg white halves onto serving platter. Add all ingredients to yolk mixture and beat until smooth and creamy. Add additional sea salt and pepper to taste. Using the back of a teaspoon, ladle the yolk mixture into egg white halves and garnish. Cover. Chill until ready to serve.

Magic eggs...they disappear.

A.W.E. – *ADD 4 oz. lump crabmeat to the yolks once beaten,
folding until just incorporated
OR – ADD a little horseradish
OR – ADD pesto to the egg mixture
before filling egg halves
OR – ADD wasabi and a few black sesame seeds*

FACT: *For the perfect hard-boiled egg (without discoloration of the yolk),
place eggs in a pot and cover with cold water.
Bring to a rapid boil, uncovered.
Remove from heat and cover (no peeking) for 15 minutes.
Place in cold water with ice until eggs are cool to the touch.
*note: To assure yolks are always in the middle of the egg white,
remove them from their egg crates and lay them on their side
24 hours before boiling them.*

NO-BONES BUFFALO CHICKEN DIP

8 oz. cream cheese
8 oz. sour cream
8 oz. blue cheese dressing
8 oz. blue cheese, crumbled
2-½ cups of cooked chicken, finely chopped
⅓ cup hot sauce
8 oz. sharp cheddar, or tex-mex cheese, shredded

Preheat oven to 350 degrees

Mix all ingredients in a bowl. Place in a greased (with coconut oil), glass 8" x 8" glass baking dish, and bake for 25 minutes, covered with parchment paper-lined foil. Uncover and cook an additional 5 minutes. Serve with celery sticks.

Lick-your-fingers good.

A.W.E. – *OMIT blue cheese dressing and crumbles,
and ADD 16 oz. sour cream and 8 oz. ranch dressing
OR – OMIT celery and serve in endive boats (individual endive leaves)
OR – OMIT chicken and ADD cooked shrimp*

FACT: *Chicken is a great source of B6, protein, niacin and selenium.*

PETE'S SMOKIN' FISH DIP

16 oz. cream cheese, softened
8 oz. sour cream
1-½ cups smoked fish (of your choice), shredded
4 scallions, chopped
2 medium shallots, chopped (or 1 large shallot)
2 Tbsps. horseradish
sea salt and freshly ground black pepper
celery sticks for serving

Mix all ingredients. Chill before serving. Serve with celery sticks.

Watch out for double-dippers !

A.W.E. – *ADD 1 fresh jalapeño pepper, diced*
(with or without ribs & seeds)
OR – for some smoky heat, ADD a chipotle pepper, diced
(with or without ribs & seeds)

FACT: *Smoking to preserve fish,*
is an age-old method practiced in
Scandinavia, Great Britain, and other Northern European countries.

CREAM CHEESE TIDBITS

- Philadelphia brand cream cheese is one of the oldest American packaged foods.

- It went on sale (in its protective wrapper) in 1885.

SAUSAGE 'N PEPPER PIE

1 cup sausage (no sugar added), cooked, crumbled
1-¼ cups jarlsberg cheese (or swiss), shredded
1-¼ cups parmesan cheese, shredded
½ cup green bell pepper, finely chopped
1 cup yellow onion, coarsely chopped
1 cup Mayonnaise (pg. 7)
freshly ground black pepper to taste
celery slices, or widely sliced bell peppers, as "dippers"

Preheat oven to 325 degrees

In a pan, cook crumbled sausage until no longer pink. Remove from heat, and drain. Place sausage in a bowl and add all ingredients. Stir well. Place mixture in a greased (with coconut oil), 8" x 8" glass baking dish (or round glass pie dish). Bake uncovered until top is golden brown, approximately 35 to 45 minutes. Serve hot with celery sticks or pepper slices, for that sausage-onion-pepper taste, you love so much.

One. Dip. Two. Dip.

A.W.E. – *OMIT crumbled sausage making it an onion pie.*
Cook up some crispy sausage patties, to serve it on.

FACT: *Red bell peppers are*
3x higher than green bell peppers in vitamin C,
and 11x higher in beta carotene.

BUBBLIN' CRAB DIP

1 to 1-¼ lbs. fresh crab meat
4 oz. cream cheese, softened
¼ cup sour cream
½ cup cheddar cheese, shredded
½ cup parmesan cheese, grated
¼ cup Mayonnaise (pg. 7)
2 green onions, finely chopped
1 Tbsp. fresh lemon juice
½ cup pork rinds, finely crushed (pg. 28)

Preheat oven to 350 degrees

Combine all ingredients except for pork rinds, mixing well. Pour mixture into a greased (with grape seed oil) 8" x 8" glass baking dish. Sprinkle top with crushed pork rinds and bake uncovered, 20 to 25 minutes or until bubbly. Serve on your choice of "Faux" Cracker (pg. 4).

Bubble. Bubble. It's no trouble !

A.W.E. – *ADD artichoke hearts*

FACT: *Pork rinds, as well as nuts, are the only "junk food" you can buy in the chip aisle, and eat guilt-free.*

CHILL-E CRAB DIP

8 oz. cream cheese, softened
½ cup No Skippin' Shrimpin' (Cocktail Sauce, pg.10)
1 large can crabmeat
Watch out! Some canned crab has sugar added.
sea salt and freshly ground black pepper

Combine cream cheese and cocktail sauce. Mix well. Fold in crab meat.
Add salt and pepper to taste. Refrigerate at least one hour before serving.

Don't crowd the crab.

A.W.E. – *ADD a few chopped scallions and shallots*
OR – ADD fresh chopped jalapeño's and garlic
OR – ADD diced cooked shrimp and warm it up
OR – serve it hot but ADD a few finely crushed pork rinds on the top for crunch

FACT: *Crabs are found in ALL of the world's oceans.*
Crabs live in fresh water and on land,
particularly in tropical regions.

HOLY GUACAMOLE!

8 ripened avocados, peeled, pitted and diced
½ red onion, diced
4 plum tomatoes, juiced, seeded, and diced
2 Tbsps. fresh cilantro (or more)
½ tsp. garlic powder
½ tsp. chipotle powder
sea salt and freshly ground black pepper
½ fresh lime, juiced

In a mixing bowl, mash avocado into paste, and add red onion. Mix in tomatoes, cilantro, garlic, and chipotle powder, stirring well. Season with salt and pepper to taste. Add lime juice and mix right before serving. Serve on your choice of Faux Cracker (pg. 4) or fresh cut veggies like peppers or celery (or put it on top of your favorite cooked proteins).

Avocado heaven.

A.W.E. – *OMIT chipotle powder (a smoky flavor),
and ADD minced fresh jalapeño peppers, with or without ribs & seeds.
Choose your heat.*

FACT: *Avocado is heart healthy!
To ripen an avocado, place it in a brown paper bag for 2 to 5 days.
To store a ripened avocado, keep it refrigerated.
Always wash the skin before peeling.
Lime juice helps guacamole keep its vibrant, avocado-green color.*

LET YOUR PIGGY ROLL

this recipe requires freezing before use

Nitrate-free ham slices
8 oz. cream cheese, softened
1 medium yellow onion, minced
plastic wrap

Combine softened cream cheese with minced onion. Mix well. Spread cream cheese evenly down entire length of ham slices. Starting at one end, roll the ham into a log. Place ham roll-ups in plastic wrap, sealing tightly. Freeze. Remove ham roll-up approximately ten minutes before serving. Cut across ham rolls, to create mini-pinwheels.

Ham it up!

A.W.E. – *OMIT cream cheese and ADD roasted garlic, spinach, and brie cheese*
OR – OMIT ham and ADD turkey
OR – ADD a raw, trimmed asparagus spear, or pickle to add crunch

FACT: *Cream cheese was developed in 1872 in New York, made from milk and heavy cream.*

BAKED BRIE

*this recipe requires the making of Dough (pg. 26)
prior to preparation

1 brie wheel
dough
1 Tbsp. butter, melted
sweetener of your choice
dash of lemon juice
3 granny smith apples, sliced (to serve on)

Preheat oven to 400 degrees

Roll dough out large enough to cover brie wheel. Place the brie in the center of the dough, carefully folding the edges of the dough toward top. Pull off any excess dough, and flatten the top as you work. *(Remember- you are actually working on the bottom of the cheese.)* Dough is moist and will likely tear when bent this way. Fill in any spaces or holes. Carefully flip the dough crusted wheel over. Place in a greased (with grape seed oil) glass 8" x 8" baking dish. *(*option: shape a small design out of the leftover dough, and affix it to the top of the wheel, with a dab of melted butter).* Bake 16 to 20 minutes, or until top is a light golden brown. Remove from oven, and allow to sit in baking dish for 10 minutes. Do not cut into the baked brie too soon, or all of your cheese will ooze out. Move brie to a serving platter (with a lip), and place apple slices around the perimeter.

Ooooey-gooooey goodness.

A.W.E. – *ADD fresh berries with a little sweetener, OR fruit-only sweetened jelly on the dough, before placing brie in its center.*

FACT: *The most desirable portion on a wedge of Brie is the tip.
Removing the tip is referred to as
"pointing the Brie," and is regarded as a no-no!*

EAT-YOUR-SPINACH SQUARES

1 (10 oz.) package of frozen chopped spinach (thawed & drained)
4 large eggs, beaten
½ cup sour cream
Sea salt and freshly ground black pepper
1 tsp. minced garlic
1 cup of cheddar cheese, shredded

Preheat oven to 400 degrees

Grease (with grape seed oil) an 8" x 8" glass baking dish. In a mixing bowl, combine all ingredients. Pour into baking dish. Bake for 15 minutes. Turn oven off, leaving the dish inside for an additional 10 to 15 minutes. Cut into bite-size pieces (or larger pieces, if you're serving them as a meal). Serve hot.

Spinach².

A.W.E. – *ADD your favorite cheese*
OR – ADD crumbled cooked sausage or bacon

FACT: *The more prominent the CHALAZA,*
(the white ropy strand attached to the yolk),
the fresher the egg.

JALAPEÑO CHEESE 'EMS

½ stick of butter (4 oz.)
1 medium onion, finely diced
2 Tbsps. minced garlic
16 oz. cream cheese, softened
1 tsp. sea salt
1 tsp. freshly ground black pepper
3 chicken breasts, cooked and finely diced (or shredded)
30 jalapeño peppers
30 strips bacon
30 toothpicks
grape seed oil

Preheat oven to 350 degrees

Melt butter in sauté pan, adding onions and cooking until translucent. Add garlic. Sauté until edges of onion turn brown. In a large bowl add onions and garlic to the softened cream cheese, stirring well. Add cooked chicken, salt, and pepper, mixing thoroughly. Slit jalapeño peppers down one side, leaving the tops and stems on. Remove all of the seeds and ribs from inside the peppers. Once cleaned, pressing on the top and bottom of the pepper (to "open" it), fill the jalapeño with the cream cheese mixture. Once filled, wrap each pepper with one slice of bacon. Secure bacon with a toothpick through the middle of the pepper. Place in the bottom of a large, glass baking dish (10" x 14"), (greased with grape seed oil). Bake 30 minutes, or until bacon is cooked.

Some like it hot.

A.W.E. – *for a hot and spicy popper, do NOT remove ALL of the seeds and ribs of the jalapeño peppers*

FACT: *Chipotle peppers are jalapeño peppers that have been smoked and dried.*

STUFFED "MATOES"

12 plum tomatoes
24 fresh basil leaves
1 block, fresh mozzarella cheese

Preheat oven to 350 degrees
OR
Preheat grill to medium-low

note: this recipe may also be served cold without heating

Cut plum tomatoes in half width-wise. Empty seeds and juice forming a "cup." Cut off just enough of the bottom of each tomato half, so that they easily sit flat. Put a whole basil leaf in bottom of each tomato half. Cut mozzarella into small cubes (to fit into tomato cup). Insert cheese to sit on top of basil leaf. *If cooking on a grill*, it's easiest to use a vegetable cage, or iron skillet. *If cooking in the oven*, place in a glass baking dish. Cook for 15 to 20 minutes. It's done when the cheese is bubbly and delicious.

Don't drop 'em ...pop 'em .

A.W.E. – *OMIT the basil and mozzarella cheese and*
ADD sautéed onions and goat cheese
OR – serve with balsamic vinegar, or a balsamic glaze drizzled on top
OR – use campari tomatoes instead of plum tomatoes.
(*note: campari tomatoes are sweet and noted for their juiciness,
low acidity and lack of a mealy texture. They are bigger than cherry tomatoes,
but smaller than plum tomatoes.)

FACT: *Nightshade vegetables grow at night, and contain solanine*
(a glucoalkaloid), that interferes with the body's ability to absorb calcium.
Nightshades include: eggplants, red and green bell peppers, tomatoes, tomatillos, hot
peppers, pimento, paprika, fennel, gogi berries, cherries, tobacco and white potato. Soy
sauce (manufactured in the U.S.), is made with GMO
(Genetically Modified) soy beans, and diluted with the nightshade petunia.
Studies are beginning to link nightshade ingestion with a negative impact on people
suffering with: arthritis, alzheimer's, chronic fatigue, cancer, eczema, depression,
wheat and dairy sensitivities, memory loss, migraines,
parkinson's, and osteoporosis- to name a few.

"FAUX" SUSHI

*this recipe requires preparation and refrigeration before use

2 cups tuna, sushi-grade, cubed
2 avocados, cubed
½ cup japanese mayonnaise
1 tsp. wasabi
2 small cucumbers, peeled, sliced ¼"
(if you use an english cucumbers- leave skins on)
nori (seaweed) flakes (as garnish)
black sesame seeds (as garnish)

Combine mayonnaise, and wasabi. Mix well. Add tuna, and avocado cubes and toss lightly. Refrigerate a minimum of 30 minutes. Spoon mixture on top of sliced cucumber. Garnish with nori and sesame seeds. For those who like it "spicy," add a dab of wasabi to the top before serving.

Spicy. No ricey.

A.W.E. – *ADD a dab of fish roe (caviar) as a garnish*
OR – *OMIT dried nori flakes and ADD seaweed salad OR sesame seeds*

FACT: *Wasabi is a member of the brassicaceae family,*
which includes mustard, horseradish, and cabbages.
Wasabi is also known as Japanese horseradish.

"COOL-AS-A-CUCUMBA" DIP

2 cups sour cream (or Greek yogurt)
1 large cucumber, peeled and diced
(english cucumbers have fewer seeds,
helping dip remain less watery)
½ tsp. sea salt (or more to personal taste)
2 Tbsps. olive oil
2 cloves garlic, minced
2 Tbsps. white vinegar
fresh dill, chopped (as garnish)

Place all ingredients (except for dill), into a food processor. Pulse until *just* blended. Add additional salt to taste. Pour into serving bowl and refrigerate for a minimum of 1 hour. Garnish with dill. Serve with pepperoni or salami crisps, celery sticks or cucumber slices.

Put up your cukes!

A.W.E. *– ADD cooked, diced shrimp*
OR – OMIT dill and ADD parsley & chives

FACT: *Do not store cucumbers near fruit.*
Fruits emit ethylene gas (which enhances ripening),
causing cucumbers to rot more quickly.

CUCUMBER TIDBIT

- The term "cool as a cucumber," is derived from the cucumber's ability to cool the temperature of the blood when eaten. Applied topically, cucumber really does cool the blood and ease facial swelling, which is the reason they are so popular in facial and eye regiments.

STRAWBERRY SALSA

1 pint strawberries, coarsely chopped
2 ripened avocados, diced
¼ cup fresh cilantro, finely chopped
¼ cup fresh lime, or lemon juice
2 Tbsps. olive oil
½ red bell pepper, finely chopped
1 small red onion, finely chopped
2 jalapeño peppers, ribs and seeds removed, finely chopped

Mix all ingredients in a small bowl. Cover and refrigerate until serving. Do not make this salsa too far ahead of time, as diced avocado will discolor. Serve on cucumber rounds. Try using this salsa as a topping for grilled fish or chicken.

Dollops all around.

A.W.E. *– for a spicier salsa allow a few seeds and ribs to remain inside the jalapeño peppers*

FACT: *Strawberries are rich in nitrate, and increase blood flow, which increases oxygen to your muscles.*

STRAWBERRY TIDBITS

- Strawberries are the first fruit to ripen in the spring.

- Strawberries are a member of the rose family.

- Strawberries are the only fruit with seeds on the outside (about 200 on a single berry).

- 94% of U.S. households consume strawberries.

CLAMS CASINO

24 Little Neck clams, completely closed
note: if they are open, it means they are bad!
8 strips bacon, cut into 1" pieces
(you need enough bacon to make 24, 1-½" pieces)
1 green OR red bell pepper, minced
3 Tbsps. butter
2 shallots, minced

Preheat oven to 350 degrees

Rinse clams in cold water. Shuck clams (see FACT). Leave the clam and its juice on one side of the shell. Discard the remaining shell half. Cook bacon half way through. Drain and cut bacon into "clam" size pieces. Mince pepper and shallots, and mix together. To each clam, add the shallot/pepper mixture, a piece of bacon, and finally a tiny pat of butter. Bake 25 to 35 minutes, or until bacon is thoroughly cooked.

BET you'll love 'em!

A.W.E. – *ADD a few finely crushed pork rinds (pg. 28),
topped with butter for a little "crunch"*

FACT: *Shucking a clam isn't as hard as you might think.
First, place them in the freezer for five minutes
to loosen their hold on the shell.
Work over an empty bowl to collect any juice.
Hold the clam in your hand with the shell hinge toward your palm.
Insert a thin, dull knife (never a sharp one) between both shell sides.
Work the knife around so you can cut through the hinge.
Open the shell, and slide the knife between the clam, and the top of its shell.
Detach the clam by sliding the knife between
the top and the bottom of its shell.*

PARTY PLEASIN' PINWHEELS

8 oz. cream cheese, softened
1 Tbsp. prepared horseradish
½ cup sharp cheddar cheese, shredded
sea salt and freshly ground black pepper to taste
1 lb. roast beef, sliced

option: 1 cup lettuce (your choice), finely shredded

Mix cream cheese, horseradish, cheddar cheese, salt, and pepper in a bowl. Overlap two slices of roast beef (at one end of each), sprinkling the top and bottom lightly with salt and pepper. Apply a ⅛ - ¼" layer of the cream cheese mixture, across the roast beef. Sprinkle the optional lettuce on top of cream cheese. Starting at one end of roast beef, roll it up until you have formed a "log." Wrap them up and place in the freezer for 15 minutes. Remove immediately and cut into ½" pieces. Place the mini-pinwheels on their sides directly onto your serving tray.

The wheels on the table go...

A.W.E. – *OMIT roast beef, horseradish and cheddar cheese,
and ADD 1 finely chopped scallion to the cream cheese
OR – OMIT roast beef, cheddar, and horseradish and
ADD salted turkey slices and thin strips (use a vegetable peeler)
of granny smith apple (cored and peeled), on top of cream cheese*

FACT: *Cream cheese is high in vitamin A.
If you run low on butter, cream cheese may be successfully used
as a partial replacement in cake recipes.
Use the ratio of 2:1 (2 parts cream cheese to 1 part butter)
to replace original butter amounts
dictated in your recipe.*

More Helpful Hints and Ideas

- **CRUDITE**: Cut your favorite veggies and place them on a platter served with one of your favorite dips, or ours!

- **CHEESE Plate**: Always a hit. Toothpicks make things easy.

- **SHRIMP COCKTAIL**: Who doesn't like shrimp? Cooked shrimp served with No Skimpin' Shrimpin' (Cocktail Sauce, pg. 10).

- **CRACKERS**: Make your own (pgs. 3 & 4).

- **GRILLED VEGGIES** (pg. 138), for an antipasto platter.

- **CAULIFLOWER POPCORN:** Break head into small florets. Cover with grape seed oil & garlic salt. Bake 400 for 16 to 18 minutes. Sprinkle with grated cheese while hot.

- **FRUIT SKEWERS:** Alternate blackberries or strawberries, a basil leaf, and mozzarella cheese, on a wooden skewer. OR alternate raspberries and fresh mint leaves, with mozzarella balls or cubes.

- **GOAT CHEESE:** Roll balls of cheese in your favorite spices.

- **ANTIPASTO SKEWERS:** olives, cheeses, artichokes, meats, peppers, or veggies. Let your imagination run wild.

- **MINI BURGERS:** Serve with lettuce, onion, pickle, tomato, and a toothpick. Make your favorite burgers into minis!

- **PEPPERS 'N RICOTTA:** 2 red peppers, 1 cup ricotta, a little fresh garlic, salt & pepper in a blender. Pulse till well mixed. Dip away.

SOUPS

- **Cheesy Broccoli Soup**
- **Easy Escarole Soup**
- **Roasted "Mato" Soup**
- **Pot-'O-Veggie Soup**
- **Crowded Clam Soup**
- **Mexican Hat Soup**
- **Creamy Cauliflower Soup**
- **There's – Fun – In Onion Soup**
- **Cheesy, Creamy, Zucchini Soup**
- **Broccoli-Rabé 'N Sausage Soup**

Savory Soups
Welcome the Warmth of Health

**"The part can never be well,
unless
the whole is well."**

Plato
Greek Philosopher
427 – 347 B.C.

CHEESY BROCCOLI SOUP

1 head broccoli, finely chopped
3 Tbsps. butter
½ yellow onion, chopped
1-½ Tbsps. coconut flour
1-½ Tbsps. chickpea flour
½ tsp. dried ground thyme
½ tsp. garlic powder
½ tsp. sea salt
⅛ tsp. freshly ground black pepper
2 cups beef stock or broth
2 cups heavy cream
2 cups sharp cheddar cheese, finely shredded

note: consider doubling...this soup disappears!

Place chopped broccoli into small pot of water and boil uncovered until tender (about 20 minutes). Drain and set aside. In a small sauté pan cook onion in butter over medium heat, until tender. Blend in coconut flour, chickpea flour, and all seasonings, stirring constantly. Cook 2 to 3 minutes. Add beef stock a little at a time, stirring until thick and smooth. Remove from heat. Pull out a few tablespoons of broccoli florets. Mince finely and set aside. Ladle into a table-top blender; the cooked broccoli (not including the finely minced portion), the onion mixture, and some heavy cream in small batches, and puree. Place puree into a medium soup pot. Continue blending until all broccoli, heavy cream, and onion mixtures have been pureed. Place soup pot on low heat. Add cheddar cheese and minced broccoli florets. Stir occasionally until all cheese is melted. Do NOT boil! Remove from heat and serve immediately.

Slurp your cheese.

A.W.E. – *OMIT the step that minces a few tablespoons of florets,*
if you want the soup to have a creamier texture
OR – use cauliflower instead of broccoli

FACT: *Broccoli is rich in vitamins A & C, folate, and iron.*
Choose broccoli that has dark green; purplish-green; or blue-green colored florets, as they are higher in beta-carotene and vitamin C.

EASY ESCAROLE SOUP

32 oz. chicken broth
1 head escarole, cleaned (chopped into bite-size pieces)
1 tsp. dried thyme
1 tsp. dried oregano
1 tsp. dried basil
1 tsp. garlic powder
½ tsp. paprika
½ tsp. freshly ground black pepper
2 eggs
optional garnish: grated parmesan, asiago, or locatelli cheese

To a large pot add chicken broth and all of the ingredients *except* for the eggs. Cover and simmer on low for 1 to 1-½ hours, stirring occasionally. Uncover and add chopped escarole. Simmer an additional 25 minutes. In a small bowl beat two eggs. Stirring soup constantly, pour the beaten eggs slowly into pot. Continue cooking for three more minutes. Serve immediately. *garnish with grated cheese, immediately before serving.*

No slurping.

A.W.E. – *ADD homemade "mini" meatballs*
OR – ADD cooked sausage pieces and garlic

FACT: *Escarole has a bold, almost bitter flavor.*
The most tender leaves are the inner-most ones.
Escarole is rich in folate, vitamins A & C, and calcium.

ROASTED "MATO" SOUP

2 lbs. plum tomatoes
¼ medium red onion, chopped
1 Tbsp. dried oregano
3 fresh basil leaves, finely chopped
6 tsps. garlic, minced
2 Tbsps. balsamic vinegar
2 Tbsps. grape seed or peanut oil
sea salt and freshly ground black pepper
2 cups chicken broth
garnish with ¼ cup shaved or grated parmesan cheese

Preheat oven to 375 degrees

Wash and cut tomatoes lengthwise and put them, face up, in the bottom of a glass baking dish. Place onion, oregano, basil, and garlic on top of tomatoes. Drizzle vinegar and oil on top of everything. Season them with salt and pepper to taste. Bake for 45 minutes. Allow them to cool enough, to handle comfortably. Peel the skin from tomatoes and place them in a blender or food processor. Puree tomatoes in small batches, while adding chicken broth, a little at a time. Place puree in small soup pot. Continue process until all of the tomatoes and broth have been pureed. Reheat soup. Garnish with grated cheese.

Roasty toasty.

A.W.E. – *ADD cubes of fresh mozzarella cheese (or shredded cheese),*
on top of hot soup
OR – ADD ¾ cup heavy cream to make a creamy tomato soup
OR – ADD chopped fresh spinach to soup with all other ingredients
OR – ADD cooked sea scallops or cooked cubed beef

FACT: *Tomato is rich in vitamins C & A, and lycopene,*
and are powerful anti-oxidants.
Leave them on your countertop at room temperature.
Don't chill your "matoes."

POT-'O-VEGGIE SOUP

4 Tbsps. butter
1-½ cups green beans, cut bite-size
2 cups leeks (white part only), chopped
1 red bell pepper, chopped
4 celery stalks, diced
2 Tbsps. fresh garlic, finely minced
2 yellow squash, diced
2 cups fresh spinach
3 quarts chicken or vegetable broth
2 cups water
4 cups tomatoes, seeded, chopped
¼ cup fresh parsley, chopped
¼ cup fresh basil, chopped
sea salt and freshly ground black pepper

Add butter to a large skillet and sauté green beans, leeks, red pepper, and celery for 8 minutes. Add garlic, cooking an additional 5 minutes. Stir often. Place sautéed veggies into a large pot, and add squash, spinach, broth, water, tomatoes, parsley, basil, salt, and pepper to taste. Simmer covered, on low heat for a minimum of 1 hour.

Make your mother proud.
Eat ALL of your veggies !

A.W.E. – *ADD broccoli florets*
OR – substitute your favorite onion for leeks
OR – ADD a few shrimp at the end of the simmer
OR – puree soup, and ADD a little cream

FACT: *China is the leading cultivator of vegetables,*
with top productions in:
onions, lettuce, broccoli, tomatoes, and cabbage.

CROWDED CLAM SOUP

½ cup water
4 cloves garlic, minced
1 stalk celery, chopped
½ yellow onion, minced
1 tsp. sea salt
⅛ tsp. freshly ground white pepper
2 cups zucchini, peeled and cubed
(as a "potato" substitute)
1 cup heavy cream
1 cup whole milk
1 can (6-½ or 8 oz.) clams, chopped or minced
1 cup clam juice
1 Tbsp. butter

In medium saucepan heat water, garlic, celery, onion, salt, and pepper to a boil. Add cubed zucchini. Reduce heat to simmer. Cook ingredients for 10 to 12 minutes. Zucchini should still be firm. Add additional water if needed, 1 Tbsp. at a time. Add heavy cream, milk, clams, clam juice, and butter. Add additional salt and pepper to personal taste. Cook soup for an additional 5 to 10 minutes, or until thoroughly heated.

Crammin' the clams-in.

A.W.E. – *ADD cooked, cubed, spicy sausage for a kick*
OR – *OMIT yellow onion, and ADD chopped leeks*

FACT: *Never store clams in water or ice.*
Immersion in cold will cause them to die.
Store covered with a damp paper towel in the refrigerator.

MEXICAN HAT SOUP

4 boneless, skinless chicken breasts
8 cups of chicken broth
2 Tbsps. butter
1-½ cups yellow onion, chopped
2 cloves garlic, minced
2 stalks celery (including leafy tops), diced
2 jalapeño peppers, diced (remove ribs & seeds for less "heat")
1 green bell pepper, diced
3 large tomatoes, diced
2 Tbsps. fresh cilantro, chopped
sea salt and freshly ground black pepper to taste
2 tsps. red chili powder
1 tsp. cumin
1 Tbsp. dried oregano
½ lime, juiced
1 cup heavy cream
sour cream, (as garnish)
black olives, chopped (as garnish)
avocado, diced (as garnish)

Place chicken breasts and chicken broth in pot and bring to boil on high heat. As chicken cooks, dice your vegetables. Once boiling, reduce broth to simmer for 10 to 12 minutes, or until no pink remains in chicken. Remove chicken. Reserve stock. Return empty pot to stove and melt butter, adding onions and garlic. Cook until tender. Add green pepper, jalapeño peppers, and celery, also cooking until tender. Add tomatoes, salt, pepper, chili powder, cumin, oregano, and cilantro. Cover, and cook for an additional 10 minutes. Pour chicken broth back into pot, and using a hand-held blender, liquefy the soup (or use a regular blender, and puree the broth with the veggies). Cut chicken meat into bite-size chunks, long strips, or shred it, and add to puree. On low, allow soup to re-heat for 10 minutes then add your heavy cream, stirring well. Lastly, add lime juice. Serve hot and garnish with a dollop of sour cream, black olives, and avocado.

No hat-head.

A.W.E. – *ADD cooked, shrimp, swordfish, mahi-mahi, or shredded skirt steak OR – OMIT chicken and ADD sausage*

FACT: *Celery is a natural diuretic.*
Buy ORGANIC whenever possible.

8 REASONS TO EAT ORGANIC FOODS:

- They reduce the toxic load to your body

- They help protect future generations

- They reduce off-farm pollution

- They build healthy soils

- They taste better and offer truer flavors

- You assist family farmers of all sizes

- You avoid GMO's in your food

- You eat locally

CREAMY CAULIFLOWER SOUP

1 head of cauliflower, chopped
½ cup celery, chopped
1 small yellow onion, chopped
1-½ cups water
3 Tbsps. butter
1-½ Tbsps. coconut flour
1-½ Tbsps. chickpea flour
1 can coconut milk (14 oz.)
1-¼ tsps. sea salt
¼ tsp. freshly ground black pepper
(white pepper may be substituted so you don't see it in the soup)
½ tsp. curry powder
1 cup heavy cream

Cover and simmer together: cauliflower, celery and onion in water for 20 minutes or until very tender. Puree mixture in pot with a hand blender, setting aside when done. Heat butter in a small soup pot over medium heat. Blend in coconut and chickpea flours, stirring constantly for about 1 minute. Add coconut milk slowly, stirring until smooth, reduce heat to medium-low. Stir milk mixture into puree: with salt, pepper, curry, and heavy cream. Stir occasionally until hot, but do not boil! Serve immediately.

Good golly, cauli !

A.W.E. – *OMIT coconut milk and curry, and INCREASE heavy cream to 2-½ cups, and ADD 2 cups of shredded cheddar cheese*

FACT: *Cauliflower may resemble broccoli, but it is less dense, cooks faster, and has a milder taste.*

THERE'S-FUN-IN ONION SOUP

9 Tbsps. butter
10 vidalia onions
1 Tbsp. balsamic vinegar
1 tsp. coconut oil
5 or 6 beef bones (with marrow)
2 cloves garlic, minced, crushed
3 quarts beef stock
2 cups water
6 sprigs of fresh thyme
1 bay leaf
½ tsp. dry mustard
sea salt and freshly ground black pepper

Place 8 Tbsps. of butter (reserving 1 Tbsp.) in a large pot, set to low heat. Add onions and sauté, *slowly* for an hour. Add balsamic vinegar, continue cooking for fifteen minutes. Using a slotted spoon, remove onions from pot. Add coconut oil, and 1 Tbsp. butter to the pot over medium heat, and add beef bones. Cook until beef bones are browned, and then add onion back to pot. Add garlic, stock, water, thyme, bay leaf, dry mustard, salt, and pepper to personal taste. Bring to boil. Reduce heat, cover, and simmer 45 minutes. Uncover and remove all beef bones. Serve hot.

O.M.M.G.
Oh, mmmmm, mmmmm, goodness.

A.W.E. – *ADD your favorite browned beef*

FACT: *To store fresh sprigs of thyme,
stand them in a glass of water in your refrigerator.*

CHEESY, CREAMY, ZUCCHINI SOUP

2 large yellow onions, chopped
3 celery stalks, chopped
8 Tbsps. butter
5 Tbsps. coconut flour
1-½ tsps. thyme, dried
freshly ground black pepper to taste
32 oz. beef broth or stock
6 to 8 cups zucchini, peeled, and chopped
(about 7 medium-size zucchinis)
2 cups cheddar cheese (shredded or chopped)
½ cup heavy cream
sea salt

Sauté onion and celery in half of the butter until translucent not browned. Add thyme, pepper and remaining butter and coconut flour. Mix and cook on low for about 3 minutes stirring constantly. Slowly add beef broth, stirring until bubbling. Add zucchini and cook on low until soft (20 to 25 minutes). Remove from heat. Puree all ingredients until smooth. Return back to heat and add cheese. Do not boil. Heat until all the cheese is melted. Salt to taste. Add cream, remove from heat, and serve immediately.

Cheesey...pleasey.

A.W.E. – *for a chunkier version, ADD cooked, crumbled sausage*

FACT: *Zucchini is tender and tasty when young,
but tasteless when large and overgrown.
When selecting the perfect zucchini, choose ones that are
firm and heavy for their size.*

BROCCOLI-RABÉ 'N SAUSAGE SOUP

1 large package hot sausage
1 bunch broccoli-rabé
washed and torn into bite-size pieces
(plus water to boil it in)
1 Tbsp. butter
1 sweet onion, chopped
2 cloves fresh garlic, chopped
3 quarts chicken broth
2 cups water (for soup)
3 eggs (beaten separately)

Preheat oven to 375 degrees

Bake sausage for 40 minutes. When done, cut into bite-size pieces and set aside. Fill a medium size pot halfway with water and bring to a boil. Remove and discard the large, thick stems only, from the broccoli-rabé. Cut remaining stems and leaves into bite size pieces and add to the boiling water. Boil until broccoli-rabé turns bright green (this will only take a few minutes), then drain completely and set aside. In a large pot over medium heat, add butter, and onions. Sauté until transparent. Add garlic, cooking an additional 3 minutes stirring continuously. Add chicken broth, water, broccoli-rabé, and cooked sausage pieces. Reduce heat to low. Cover and simmer 45 minutes. Remove cover. Return heat to medium high, while constantly stirring pot, add 1 beaten egg at a time, to create strings of egg. Serve immediately.

Rabé 'n the soup.

A.W.E. – *ADD a little green bell pepper for everyone's favorite...*
sausage and peppers

FACT: *Broccoli-rabé is also known as rapini.*
and is high in vitamins A, C, K, potassium, calcium, and iron.

More Helpful Hints and Ideas

- **Homemade Soups are waiting:** Tomato & Basil; New England Clam; Seafood Chowder; Turkey Chili; Chicken; Veal Goulash; Cream of Asparagus; Italian Sausage; Cream of Mushroom; Jambalaya; Italian Wedding; Cream of Chicken; Beef Gumbo; Cream of Celery; Chicken Vegetable; Cream of Tomato; Eggplant; Vegetable Beef; Sausage Gumbo. Quick! Find a pot.

- **Americans eat 10 BILLION bowls of soup every year.**

- **Clear Broth (consommé):** was created by the royal chefs of a French King in the 1700's, who insisted they develop a soup that he could see his reflection in.

- **Hot soups have a "steam" benefit:** while sipping and breathing in the steam from hot soup, it helps to clear head congestion (the same way a hot shower does).

- **Soup:** is a mainstay in the everyday diet of most cultures. It is believed to have been one of the earliest foods prepared, as it could be made with anything (including leftovers), and greatly extended simply by adding liquid. Soup may be broth-like, smooth and creamy, or chunky with proteins and vegetables.

- **Make your own Beef Broth**: 6 lbs. beef bones, roast in 400 degree oven for 45 minutes. In a large 6 quart covered pot, place 2 Tbsps. butter, 2 vidalia onions roughly chopped, an entire small bunch of thyme tied together, 5 garlic cloves smashed, 4 stalks of celery, roughly chopped. Sweat veggies on low until onions are opaque. ADD a small can of tomato paste, the roasted bones, 5 bay leaves, a few fresh peppercorns, and a handful of fresh parsley roughly chopped. Add water until pot is ¾ full. Simmer (with a lid set askew), for 5 hours, Skim as needed. Strain.

- **Cheesecloth**: wrapped around the end of a wooden spoon or spatula, makes a great way to skim off the top of soup Everything sticks to it, and it's lint-free.

SALADS

- "Mato" & Mozzarella Salad
- Eat-Your-Spinach Salad
- Cobb Salad Parfait
- Duke's Cuke Salad
- Berry Goat Cheese Salad
- Citrus Herb Salad
- B & B Salad
- Spin Your Salad
- Avocado Ranch Dressing
- Onion Vinaigrette Dressing
- Basic Balsamic Dressing

Seasoned Salads
Good Health Tossed In

**"Let food
be thy medicine,
thy medicine
shall be thy food."**

Hippocrates
Greek Physician
460 – 377 B.C.

"MATO" & MOZZARELLA SALAD

1 fresh ball mozzarella cheese, sliced
4 large heirloom tomatoes in various colors (similar to size of cheese ball)
1 large red onion, sliced
½ cup balsamic vinegar
4 Tbsps. extra virgin olive oil
sea salt and freshly ground black pepper to taste
6 to 8 fresh basil leaves, chopped (as garnish)

Cut the fresh mozzarella and tomatoes in to ¼" slices each. Arrange cheese and tomato slices on a lipped plate, alternating each. Follow the circle of the plate to form a wreath. To a skillet add the sliced onion and vinegar, cooking on low until tender. Drizzle heated onion/vinegar mixture on top of your tomato and cheese wreath. Drizzle the olive oil on top of the tomato, onion, and cheese. Add salt and pepper. Garnish with chopped basil leaves.

M. & M.'s.

A.W.E. – *ADD slices of cucumber between mozzarella cheese and tomato
to give it an extra crunch
OR – OMIT tomatoes and ADD grilled eggplant or zucchini*

FACT: *Fresh mozzarella cheese is high in water content,
and should be eaten fairly soon
after production.*

EAT-YOUR-SPINACH SALAD

1 large bunch fresh spinach
torn into bite-size pieces
½ lb. bacon, cut into bite-size pieces
1 large Portobello mushroom, sliced into bite-size pieces
½ small red onion, thinly sliced
3 tsps. dijon mustard
¼ cup red wine vinegar
sea salt and freshly ground black pepper to taste

Cook bacon pieces in pan until soft. Add mushrooms and onion, cooking until the onions are tender. Whisk mustard and vinegar together, and then add to pan. Add salt and pepper. Pour dressing over fresh spinach. Toss and serve.

Green. Warm. Good.

A.W.E. – *crumble a hard-boiled egg or goat cheese into your salad*
OR – OMIT spinach and ADD frisee

FACT: *Spinach is extremely rich in anti-oxidants,*
especially when fresh steamed or quickly boiled.
Fresh spinach loses most of its nutritional value
within a few days of picking.

COBB SALAD PARFAIT

2 small romaine hearts, leaves separated
4 eggs, hard-boiled, chopped
12 slices bacon, cooked and crumbled
1 cup sour cream
1 cup blue cheese crumbles (or swiss cheese, cubed)
1 tsp. hot sauce
sea salt and freshly ground black pepper to taste
3 avocados, mashed
½ fresh lemon, juiced
4 plum tomatoes, chopped
2 cups chicken, cooked and chopped (into bite-size pieces)
¼ cup walnuts, finely chopped

In a medium bowl, mix sour cream, blue cheese, hot sauce, salt, and pepper. In a separate bowl mash the avocados with the back of a fork. Add lemon juice and a little salt. Using a spoon place a portion of each ingredient in a small glass bowl or clear parfait cup, creating layers as follows: chopped tomato, avocado mash, chopped chicken, chopped egg, walnuts, blue cheese mixture, top with crumbled bacon pieces. Serve with whole romaine leaves...and a spoon.

Lick the cup.

A.W.E. – *OMIT chicken and ADD sliced*
OR – OMIT blue cheese and ADD your favorite cheese

FACT: *Romaine lettuce is higher in nutrients than almost
all other types of lettuce.
Varieties of Romaine include:
Sweet Romaine and Red Tipped Romaine.*

DUKE'S CUKE SALAD

6 cucumbers, peeled, and sliced thinly
1 cup sour cream
½ cup apple cider vinegar
1 tsp. xylitol sweetener
½ medium red onion, diced
½ cup fresh dill, chopped
2 Tbsps. water
sea salt and freshly ground black pepper

In a large bowl, mix all ingredients together. Cover with plastic wrap. Refrigerate until ready to serve. The longer it sits, the better it gets.

C.M.C.
Crunchy. Munchy. Cukes.

A.W.E. – *ADD 1 pint of grape tomatoes, halved*

FACT: *Dill is a great source of vitamin C, folate, potassium, and beta carotene.*

BERRY GOAT CHEESE SALAD

1 head of boston leaf lettuce (or spinach)
torn into bite-size pieces
option: may use bitter dandelion greens, or arugula
for a great contrast of flavors

8 fresh basil leaves, chopped
¼ cup balsamic vinegar
4 Tbsps. goat cheese, crumbled
½ cup olive oil (or more to personal taste)
1 pint fresh strawberries (cleaned, sliced)
sea salt and freshly ground black pepper to taste

Put lettuce leaves in large salad bowl and toss with basil. Drizzle with vinegar. Toss well. Add olive oil and mix thoroughly. Add sliced strawberries, salt, and pepper. Pile salad on serving plate and top with crumbled goat cheese.

Berry good.

A.W.E. – *OMIT strawberries and ADD diced granny smith apples*
OR – *make an appetizer, by cutting green end off berry (making it flat),*
so that strawberry sits "point" up.
Cut an "X" into tip of strawberry and stuff with goat cheese.
Sprinkle with salt, pepper and chopped basil
OR – *make a dessert by OMITTING goat cheese in the berry, and ADD*
sweetened cream cheese (with vanilla and xylitol), as a dessert

FACT: *It is important to add any vinegars or citrus juices,*
BEFORE oil, when making a salad.
Using oil first,
will prohibit the vinegars complete saturation of lettuce leaves.
Same thing applies when WASHING lettuce.
Always DRY the leaves before dressing.

CITRUS HERB SALAD

1 head of romaine lettuce (or personal favorite)
torn into bite-size pieces
1 cucumber, halved and sliced
1 bunch fresh dill, finely chopped
1 small red onion, chopped
1 block of feta cheese (water-packed is preferred)
1-½ fresh lemons, juiced
¼ cup extra virgin olive oil
sea salt and freshly ground black pepper
*option: sliced black olives

Place cleaned and dried lettuce in a salad bowl. Add cucumber slices. Add ¾ of the chopped dill and red onion. Crumble and add all the feta cheese. Squeeze lemon juice over salad. Make sure to toss until all leaves are evenly covered. Add ¼ cup olive oil (and black olives if desired). Add sea salt and pepper to taste. Sprinkle the remaining dill and onion on top before serving.

Herbalicious.

A.W.E. – *ADD grilled shrimp, chicken, steak or salmon*
OR – OMIT feta cheese and ADD goat cheese
OR – OMIT lemon juice and ADD your favorite vinegar
OR – ADD bell peppers, or grape tomatoes, for more crunch and color

FACT: *Feta cheese is either made from sheep, or goat's milk,*
and if stored correctly (in its brine),
may last up to one year in your refrigerator.

B & B SALAD
(Blue Cheese & Bacon)

2 Tbsps. red wine vinegar
¼ cup olive oil
1 Tbsp. grainy mustard
sea salt and freshly ground black pepper
1 cup blue cheese crumbles
1 avocado, peeled and sliced
12 grape tomatoes, whole or halved
8 slices bacon, cooked, crumbled
½ lb. lettuce of choice

Whisk together vinegar, oil, mustard, salt, and pepper to taste, in the bottom of your salad bowl. Add all other ingredients. Toss well, until evenly coated.

We love being blue.

A.W.E. – *ADD chopped cucumber OR blanched asparagus, for an extra crunch*

FACT: *Most blue cheese is cow's milk, but it can also be made with the milk from ewes and goats. Some popular styles of this are: Roquefort, Stilton, Gorgonzola, and Danablu.*

SPIN YOUR SALAD

Ideas to help you fan the salad flames...

- Strawberries, sautéed vidalia onions, toasted walnuts, and shredded Mozzarella cheese over mesclun greens
- Granny smith apples, sautéed vidalia onions, toasted walnuts, and shredded sharp cheddar cheese over mesclun greens
- Watercress, blue cheese, and almonds
- Use crumbled kale chips (pg. 71), for a crunch (or nuts)
- Endive, cherry tomato halves, cucumber, toasted hazelnuts
- Baby kale or watercress with bacon, garlic and shallot
- Blue cheese dressing: 1 cup of mayonnaise (pg. 7), 1 cup of buttermilk, ½ cup sour cream, 1-½ tsps. each of onion power and garlic powder, 1-½ cups blue cheese crumbles (garnish with diced tomatoes and crumbled bacon)
- Romaine and kale with eggplant, bell pepper, tomato, red onion, and shaved romano cheese
- Arugula, sun-dried tomatoes, provolone, onion, red pepper
- Greens with sliced skirt steak, red pepper, scallion, and flat -leaf parsley
- Cheeseburger salad: Romaine lettuce piled with ground beef cooked with mustard and ketchup (pg. 8), shredded sharp cheddar cheese, sliced pickles, tomatoes, and red onion
- Add things like alfalfa sprouts, cilantro, sunflower seeds, radicchio, roasted fennel, grilled red peppers, edible flowers, grilled portobello mushrooms. Try a new spin, on your old salad favorites!

Be a salad SPINNER!

A.W.E. *– Substitute your favorite salads for one of these recipes, whose ingredients make your lips go smack!*

FACT: *The name lettuce is derived from the Latin word "Latucca," which refers to the vegetable's milky juice.*
The lettuce we have today, started out as a weed growing around the Mediterranean basin. Don't store your lettuce, with your fruit in the fridge.

AVOCADO RANCH DRESSING

1 avocado, peeled, pitted and cubed
½ cup Mayonnaise (pg. 7)
½ cup sour cream
2 Tbsps. buttermilk
1-½ tsps. distilled white vinegar
1-½ tsps. red wine vinegar
¼ tsp. sea salt
⅛ tsp. garlic powder
½ tsp. dried parsley
¼ tsp. dried dill weed
¼ tsp. onion powder

note: a little bit of pure ascorbic powder (vitamin c), will delay the browning of this great dressing

Mash avocado in a bowl. Stir in mayonnaise, sour cream, buttermilk and vinegars. Stir well. Mix in all remaining ingredients. Chill before serving. Add extra buttermilk (milk, or cream), a tablespoon at a time, to create a thinner dressing (if desired). Store in an airtight container.

Addictive.

A.W.E. – *OMIT sour cream and ADD full-fat, greek yogurt*

FACT: *Avocado has the highest protein content of any fruit. There is more potassium in an avocado than there is in a banana.*

ONION VINAIGRETTE

4 scallions, finely chopped
1 Tbsp. lemon juice
¼ cup olive oil
2 tsps. dijon mustard
⅓ cup fresh parsley *OR* cilantro, finely chopped
freshly ground black pepper to taste

Combine, and whisk all ingredients in a bowl. Dress salad. Serve immediately.

Yummin' Onion.

A.W.E. – *OMIT scallions and ADD minced shallots*
OR – *drizzle a little into your egg or tuna salad*
OR – *marinate or dab a little onto chicken or shrimp before grilling*

FACT: *Choose onions that are dry and solid all over.*
Do not choose onions that have brown spots,
or that have already sprouted.

BASIC BALSAMIC DRESSING

2 Tbsps. balsamic vinegar
1 Tbsp. red wine vinegar
¾ cup olive oil
½ tsp. dijon mustard
1 tsp. onion powder
sea salt & freshly ground black pepper

Whisk vinegars together. Add oil slowly, whisking until combined. Add mustard, onion powder, salt, and pepper. Whisk well. Use immediately.

We love basics.

A.W.E. – *ADD toasted pine nuts (baked at 350 degrees for 9 minutes).*
They taste great in a balsamic dressed salad
OR – use dressing as a marinade.
It's great on steaks, pork, or even grilled veggies

FACT: *Onions should have a mild smell to them,*
even if their "taste" isn't mild.

More Helpful Hints and Ideas

- **OIL & VINEGAR Dressing**: is usually mixed 4:1, four parts oil, to one part vinegar. Start there. Tweak to your liking.

- **What can you toss in your salads?**: Peppers (yellow, green, or red); onion (white, sweet, red, green), leek, shallot, etc.); green beans; bacon crumbles; cheeses; cauliflower florets; broccoli florets; asparagus; egg; protein (fish, meat, chicken, etc.); fresh herbs (chive, parsley, basil, dill, etc.) Nuts (almonds, walnuts, pine nuts; pecans, etc.); olives, cranberries, cheeses. There are endless healthy choices.

- **Like FRISEE?** Top it with an over-easy egg and warm bacon.

- **SCALLION and SOUR CREAM Dressing**: 16 oz. sour cream; five scallions, finely chopped, 1 tsp. sea salt; ¼ tsp. pepper (more or less to your liking). Mix relentlessly with a fork, and then refrigerate. Best if made hours before first use. (**A.W.E.** - ADD 1 clove fresh garlic, minced, OR – ADD 3 Tbsps. fresh dill).

- **Don't use soap on a wooden salad bowl.** 1st time before use- saturate a paper towel with olive oil. Rub inside well. Allow to dry 24hrs.- or until dry to the touch. Before each use, rub 1 tsp. salt into bowl with a half clove of fresh garlic, or paper towel with oil. Drain immediately after use, do not use water. Polish with oil and store in a cheesecloth bag to prevent cracking of wood. Re-oil before each use.

- **Endive & Strawberry salad**: On top of endive place sliced fresh strawberries, cheddar cheese, some fresh chopped basil, a little thinly sliced red onions, and serve with basic balsamic dressing (pg. 123).

- **Arugula with Walnuts**: In a large salad bowl whisk together 3 Tbsps. full-fat Greek yogurt, 1 Tbsp. each of olive oil, fresh lemon juice, xylitol-sweetened honey, ¼ tsp. cinnamon, salt & pepper to taste. Add 8 cups of fresh arugula, ⅓ cup each- walnuts & dried, unsweetened cranberries, and 2 Tbsps. sunflower seeds.

VEGGIES

- Zucchini Mash
- Roasted Herb "Matoes"
- D. F. O. (Deep Fried Onions)
- Zucchini Boats
- No – Doubt Sprouts
- Cream 'N Spinach
- Dilly-Dilly Green Beans
- Cheese Please...Cauliflower
- Nuts for Kale
- Summer Slaw
- Broccoli Slaw
- Grilled Veggies
- Cabbage Mash
- Cheesy Asparagus
- Broccoli Cakes
- Loaded "Faux – Tatoes"

Clever Carbs
Spice up Your "Sides"

"Nothing would be more tiresome
than eating and drinking,
if God had not made them
a pleasure, as well,
as a necessity."

Voltaire
French Writer, Historian, Philosopher
1694 - 1778

ZUCCHINI MASH

6 to 8 green zucchini, cubed
3 Tbsps. butter
2 Tbsps. whole milk
¼ cup sour cream
2 Tbsps. prepared horseradish
1 garlic clove, smashed
1-½ cups cheddar cheese (or monterey jack), shredded
sea salt and freshly ground black pepper

Preheat oven to 350 degrees

Wash, and cut off ends of zucchini, and leaving the skin on, cut it into small cubes. Place cubed zucchini into a pot of water with a pinch of salt, and boil about 15 to 20 minutes, or until fork tender. Drain zucchini, and place in a large mixing bowl. Add the butter, milk, sour cream, horseradish, garlic, and only 1 cup of the cheese to the zucchini. Add salt and pepper generously, and mix well. Place mixture into casserole or glass baking dish and cover with remaining cheese. Bake uncovered for 15 minutes, or until cheese is melted, and the top is golden brown.

Feed me... zucchini.

A.W.E. – *OMIT cheddar and ADD swiss OR gorgonzola cheese
for a totally different taste
OR – ADD sautéed onions
OR – REPLACE butter with Herb Butter (pg. 11)*

FACT: *Horseradish is a member of the mustard family,
and inhibits growth of bacteria and viruses.
The bite and smell of horseradish root is almost non-existent
until it is grated, or ground.
Vinegar stops the volatile oils as the grinding,
or grating of the root begins.
The mildest versions of prepared horseradish
have vinegar added immediately upon breach of the root.*

ROASTED HERB "MATOES"

3 lbs. plum tomatoes, halved length-wise
2 Tbsps. coconut oil
6 cloves garlic, minced
¾ cup fresh basil, finely chopped
2 Tbsps. fresh rosemary, finely chopped
1 tsp. xylitol sweetener
1 tsp. sea salt
1 tsp. freshly ground black pepper

Preheat oven to 250 degrees

In a large bowl combine all ingredients. Stir gently. Arrange tomatoes, cut side up, in large glass baking dish. Bake approximately 3 hours, until wrinkled. Serve ANY temperature.

Garlic lovers unite.

A.W.E. – *crumble blue cheese OR goat cheese on top,
for the last half hour of baking*

FACT: *Black pepper is the spiciest of all peppercorns.
It helps to stimulate digestion and circulation.
Pepper should be purchased as "whole" peppercorns,
and "ground" right before use.
However, if you have a mold sensitivity,
you should avoid all pepper (and vinegars).*

D. F. O.
(Deep Fried Onions)

*note: this recipe works best with a deep fryer

vidalia onions
buttermilk
eggs
chestnut flour
sea salt and freshly ground black pepper
non-hydrogenated peanut oil (for deep frying)

Preheat oil in deep fryer to 375 degrees

Peel the onions, cutting them into ¼" thick rings. Soak onion slices in butter-milk for half an hour. Season chestnut flour with salt and pepper, and place in a shallow rimmed dish. In a separate shallow dish, beat a few eggs, seasoning with a little salt and pepper. Using a fork, remove onion from buttermilk. Allow to drain. Place onion into chestnut flour coating both sides. Dip onion into egg mixture, and re-dip into chestnut flour. Place immediately into hot oil. Only put a few onions at a time, or your oil temperature will drop too far. Cook until crisp, remove from oil and place on brown paper bags or paper towels. Once drained, place in a warm oven set to low heat (keeping oven door open slightly), until all frying is complete. Serve immediately (if there are any left).

You fryin'? We're flyin'.

A.W.E. – *OMIT egg and* DUST *with a combination of seasoned almond and coconut flours*
OR – *OMIT buttermilk and ADD milk*
OR – *fry them on your stovetop in a thick bottomed pan*

FACT: *Vidalia onions were first grown in the early 1930's near Vidalia, Georgia. The low amount of sulfur in the soil of the region, make the vidalia onion unusually sweet.*

ZUCCHINI BOATS

4 zucchini
3 tsps. fresh garlic, minced
sea salt and freshly ground black pepper
20 grape tomatoes, halved
½ cup parmesan cheese, grated
½ cup asiago cheese, grated
cast iron skillet

Preheat oven broiler

Split zucchini's down the middle, end-to-end, leaving the skin on. Place butter in a cast-iron frying pan set to medium high heat. Add garlic, stirring frequently until lightly browned. Sprinkle both sides of the zucchini with salt and pepper. Place them cut-side down in the hot pan. Cook 5 minutes. Turn the zucchini over, cooking until they are tender when pierced with a fork. Add tomatoes halves (5 per zucchini boat), and top with both cheeses. Cook for an additional two minutes. Place cast iron pan, under the broiler for 3 to 5 minutes, or until the cheese is browned and bubbly. Serve hot.

Row. Row.
Row your boat.

A.W.E. – *ADD sliced mushrooms, green peppers, and fresh basil*

FACT: *A zucchini has more potassium than a banana.*
Small to medium-size zucchinis, are much more flavorful than big ones.

NO-DOUBT SPROUTS

1-½ lbs. brussels sprouts
1 small white onion, sliced
1 lemon, juiced
sea salt and freshly ground black pepper
1-½ Tbsps. butter, melted
1-½ Tbsps. coconut oil, melted

Preheat oven to 350 degrees

Wash brussels sprouts thoroughly. Cut across the bottom of the sprouts, trimming up the ends. Place into a large glass baking dish (10" x 14" or bigger). Add onion, and sprinkle with lemon juice, salt, and pepper. Pour melted butter and coconut oil over sprouts/onions, mixing well. Arrange in a single layer. Bake 35 to 40 minutes until tender.

Shouts for sprouts !

A.W.E. *– OMIT lemon juice and INCREASE butter and oil to 2 Tbsps. each,
and ADD ¼ pound bacon cut into small pieces
OR – OMIT brussels sprouts and onion, and ADD asparagus and garlic*

FACT: *Although they look like mini cabbages,
brussels sprouts have a texture slightly denser, and milder, than cabbage.
Purchase brussels sprouts sold loosely when possible.
Choose those that are bright green in color, small in size, and firm to the touch.
Avoid those with blemished, or yellow leaves.*

CREAM 'N SPINACH

2 lbs. fresh spinach leaves
4 Tbsps. butter
sea salt and freshly ground black pepper
6 cloves garlic, minced
¼ cup onion, minced
¼ cup whole milk
1 cup heavy cream
¾ cup provolone cheese, shredded
½ cup parmesan cheese, shredded

Sauté spinach in 2 Tbsps. of the butter with salt and pepper, stirring constantly until wilted. Remove spinach, and set aside. Into same skillet add the remaining butter, garlic and onion, cooking 4 to 6 minutes. Add milk and heavy cream, and return spinach to pan, stirring continuously. Add provolone cheese, stirring until completely melted. Add parmesan cheese and additional salt and pepper to personal taste. Serve hot.

Everything's better with cream.

A.W.E. – OMIT parmesan & provolone cheeses,
and *ADD cheddar cheese*

FACT: *Fresh spinach should be crisp and dark green, with minimum stems.*
Spinach varieties are separated into two types, flat leaves,
and semi, or heavily-savoyed (crinkled) leaves.

DILLY-DILLY GREEN BEANS

2 lbs. fresh green beans, cut into 1" pieces
4 Tbsps. butter
2 shallots, minced
¼ cup lemon juice
2 Tbsps. fresh parsley, chopped
2 Tbsps. fresh dill, snipped into small pieces
sea salt and freshly ground black pepper

Bring a pot of water to a boil, then add the green beans. Cook approximately 5 to 6 minutes, until crisp-tender. Remove from heat, and drain. In the same pot, melt butter and stir in shallots. Cook approximately 3 to 4 minutes. Add beans, lemon juice, parsley, dill, salt, and pepper to taste. Stir well. Adjust salt, and pepper. Serve warm or chilled.

It's dilly...silly.

A.W.E. – *OMIT dill, and ADD garlic & bacon*
OR – OMIT lemon and dill and
ADD celery, garlic, rosemary, and basil

FACT: *Fresh dill is aromatic with feathery leaves.*
Once cut, dill droops quickly.
Using "wilted" dill, does not affect the flavor.
Dill may be kept in the refrigerator, wrapped in a damp paper towel,
or placed in a glass of water.
Dill may be frozen in an airtight container.

CHEESE PLEASE...CAULIFLOWER

1 head of cauliflower, cut into small florets
2 cups heavy cream (or half and half)
1-½ to 2 cups parmesan cheese, grated
3 oz. goat cheese, cut into small pieces
½ lb. monterey jack cheese, coarsely grated
sea salt and freshly ground black pepper to taste
*(white pepper may be substituted for black pepper,
so you don't see "flecks" in the sauce.)*

Preheat oven to 400 degrees

Mix all of the ingredients in a greased (with grape seed oil), medium-size casserole dish. Bake 20 to 30 minutes, or until cauliflower is soft, and sauce has thickened slightly. To "brown" the top, place under broiler for a few minutes. Remove and allow to sit for 10 minutes before serving.

Pass the dish.

A.W.E. – *OMIT cauliflower and ADD broccoli*

FACT: *Goat's milk has higher levels of minerals and vitamins A & B, than cow's milk.*

CHEESE TIDBITS

• The U.S. produces 25% of the world's cheese supply, approximately 9 billion pounds a year.

• Soft cheese is best cut with a wire, semi-hard and hard cheeses do best with a knife that has holes in the blade, which reduces sticking.

• Cottage cheese may be substituted for sour cream by simply pulsing it lightly in a blender.

NUTS FOR KALE

2 large bunches of organic kale,
stems and leaves coarsely chopped
3 Tbsps. grape seed oil
4 cloves fresh garlic, finely chopped
sea salt and freshly ground black pepper
1 cup walnuts, diced

Place oil in a large skillet over medium-high heat. Add garlic and sauté until soft. Add chopped kale, stirring occasionally until wilted. Season with salt and pepper to taste. Add walnuts, mixing well. Serve immediately.

You'll like it.

A.W.E. – *OMIT walnuts and ADD almonds*
OR – ADD crumbled goat cheese after wilting, and serve
over a cooked portobello mushroom cap

FACT: *Kale has more iron than beef,*
more calcium than milk,
and 10% more vitamin C than spinach.

WALNUT TIDBITS

- Walnuts are the oldest known tree food, and are harvested once a year (September through November).

- 99% of the U.S. national supply of walnuts, and ¾ of world trade walnuts come out of California.

- Walnuts are becoming well known for their healthy omega-3 fatty acid content.

SUMMER SLAW

½ small head green cabbage, finely shredded
2 Tbsps. sour cream
1 tsp. onion powder
¾ cup Mayonnaise (pg. 7)
2 tsps. celery salt
2 Tbsps. xylitol sweetener
2 Tbsps. white vinegar
½ Tbsp. dry mustard
sea salt and freshly ground black pepper

In a large bowl, combine all ingredients (except for cabbage), and mix well. Add cabbage, tossing until evenly coated. Adjustments for personal taste to salt, pepper, white vinegar, or xylitol, should be made. Cover and refrigerate for at least half an hour. Drain (if needed), mixing well immediately before serving.

Awwwww. Slawwwww.

A.W.E. *– use purple or white cabbage, instead of green*

FACT: *Cabbage is vitamin C rich.*
When choosing cabbage, make sure that the
stem area is not dry or split.

BROCCOLI SLAW

4 cups broccoli (stems only), uncooked, grated
¾ cup Mayonnaise (pg. 7)
wasabi paste (to personal taste)
juice of two limes
sea salt and freshly ground black pepper

Peel and finely grate broccoli stems. In a small bowl combine grated broccoli and all other ingredients. Mix well. Transfer to an airtight container and refrigerate for several hours (this will enhance flavors). Stir well before serving.

Go GREEN!

A.W.E. – *play with your acidity, by combining lemon & lime*
OR – ADD slivered almonds
OR – OMIT shredded broccoli and ADD shredded cauliflower
OR – ADD fresh horseradish instead of,
or in addition to, wasabi
(if you're a heat-a-holic)

FACT: *Store fresh broccoli unwashed in the refrigerator,*
in the crisper drawer. Wash immediately before using.
When buying a head of broccoli, choose one that does not have
a rubbery, or bending stem.

GRILLED VEGGIES

1 eggplant
2 zucchini
2 red bell peppers
½ cup balsamic vinegar
¼ cup non-hydrogenated peanut or grape seed oil
sea salt and freshly ground black pepper to taste

Preheat oven to 350 degrees
OR
Preheat grill to low

FOR GRILLING:

Cut both ends off of all the vegetables and slice lengthwise approximately ½"
thick. Place in zip-top plastic bag, and add all other ingredients. Marinate at least
30 minutes. Place vegetables on grill for 10 minutes turning occasionally, until
cooked through.

FOR OVEN:

Cube vegetables instead of slicing. Marinate for a minimum 30 minutes, using
the same method above. Place in a glass baking dish, and cook for 20 to 30 minutes, stirring occasionally.

Run for the grills !

A.W.E. – *ADD red onions, yellow OR orange bell pepper OR asparagus.*
These are wonderful as part of an antipasto platter.
Serve any temperature.

FACT: *Zucchini have more potassium than a banana.*
Small to medium sizes of zucchini are the most flavorful.
The flower of a zucchini is also edible.

CABBAGE MASH

note: this recipe is easiest with a food processor.
A manual potato masher may be used.

2 heads green cabbage
6 slices bacon, diced
1 stick butter (8 Tbsps.)
6 cloves fresh garlic, chopped
½ cup milk
1-½ cups sour cream
sea salt and freshly ground black pepper

Cut heads of cabbage into 8 wedges each and put them into a large pot of boiling water. Cook until fork tender. While cabbage cooks, place diced bacon in a large skillet over medium heat. When bacon is almost done, add butter and garlic, reducing heat to low. Drain cooked cabbage. If using a food processor, pulse on low. If not, mash manually. Once mashed, add milk and sour cream. Add the mashed cabbage to the skillet with butter, bacon, and garlic, mixing until thoroughly combined. Season with salt and pepper. Serve hot.

Dash for the mash.

A.W.E. – *ADD some mashed cauliflower*
OR – use purple cabbage for more color
OR – ADD horseradish (or Roasted Garlic 'N Horseradish Sauce, pg. 14)

FACT: *Cabbage is commonly used in cooking by pickling,*
steaming, stewing, sautéing, and braising.

CHEESY ASPARAGUS

1 bunch fresh asparagus, cleaned and trimmed
2 tsps. garlic powder
2 Tbsps. grape seed oil
sea salt and freshly ground black pepper
parmesan cheese, grated (as garnish)

Preheat oven to 400 degrees

Leaving asparagus whole, snap off woody ends *(see FACT below)*. Also remove leaf "points" up the length of the stalk. Rinse well. Dry spears. Place asparagus in a large glass baking dish. Sprinkle grape seed oil, garlic, salt, and pepper over them. Mix well. Bake in a single layer for 10 minutes. Turn asparagus over and cook an additional 10 minutes. Remove and sprinkle with grated cheese. Serve immediately.

Try 'em. You'll like 'em.

A.W.E. – *ADD strips of muenster, swiss, or provolone cheese, on top of asparagus after turning.*

FACT: *Asparagus is high in fiber, potassium, folate, thiamin and vitamin B6. Holding the spear at the very bottom with one hand, and in the middle of the stalk with your other hand, slowly bend the spear. The asparagus will break at the naturally occurring end of the ripened portion, and takes all the guess-work out of where to cut it.*

BROCCOLI CAKES

1 head of broccoli, cut into florets
2 egg whites
2 eggs, lightly beaten
⅓ cup parmesan cheese
1 Tbsp. coconut flour
1 Tbsp. almond flour
⅛ tsp. guar gum (pg. 220)
½ tsp. garlic powder
½ tsp. sea salt
½ tsp. freshly ground black pepper
2 Tbsps. grape seed oil
*(*optional garnish: Salsa)*

Place broccoli in a steamer basket inside a small saucepan over 1 inch of water. Bring to boil; cover and steam 4 minutes or until crisp-tender. Coarsely chop florets and set aside. In a large bowl combine: egg whites, eggs, cheese, coconut flour, almond flour, guar gum, garlic powder, salt, and pepper. Mix until thoroughly combined. Add broccoli florets, stirring until coated. Heat oil in a large ceramic-coated frying pan over medium heat. Drop broccoli batter into oil, 2 heaping tablespoons at a time, pressing down lightly to flatten. Cook in batches 3 to 4 minutes a side, or until golden brown. Drain on paper towels. Serve hot, topped with salsa.

Make no mistakes...
with broccoli cakes.

A.W.E. – *use leftover broccoli and skip the steaming step*
OR – OMIT broccoli and ADD fresh OR leftover cauliflower

FACT: *Broccoli has a strong, positive impact on our detoxification systems. It is rich in vitamins C & K, is a very good source of Vitamin A (an anti-oxidant), and is a great source of minerals.*

LOADED "FAUX-TATOES"
(Cauliflower Mash)

2 large heads cauliflower, chopped finely
8 Tbsps. butter
1 cup heavy cream
6 Tbsps. sour cream
1 cup half and half
12 strips of bacon, cooked and crumbled
6 Tbsps. fresh chives, (cut finely with scissors)
4 cups sharp cheddar cheese, shredded
sea salt and freshly ground black pepper

Preheat oven to 350 degrees

Boil cauliflower until soft. Drain and return to the pot. Using a potato masher, mash the cauliflower until smooth. Reserving 2 cups of cheese, add remaining ingredients to pot (mixing well), and add salt and pepper to personal taste. Place mixture into a large greased (with coconut oil), glass baking dish. Sprinkle the remaining cheese on top of mash. Bake 20 minutes, or until cheese is completely melted. To brown cheese, place under broiler for a few minutes.

Seconds required.

A.W.E. – *ADD as a topping to browned ground beef*

FACT: *Cauliflower is rich in vitamin C, high in fiber,
and is a good source of vitamin B6.
Cauliflower is 92% water and should feel heavy for its size.
The leaves surrounding the head should be bright green in color,
crisp, and never wilted.*

More Helpful Hints and Ideas

- **GREEN BEAN Idea**: try combining buttered green beans with mustard seeds and sliced almonds.

- **SAUERKRAUT your thing?** Sauté diced bacon and set aside to cool. Heat sauerkraut in leftover bacon fat until heated through, and add the bacon. Serve hot.

- **COMBINE**: leftover veggies that you have, with bacon, sausage, cheese, or spices in any combination that you like. Heat in a 350 degree oven until warm throughout, or cheese is melted. Remember, they're already cooked, so it won't take long.

- **EGGPLANT Idea**: double dip sliced eggplant in egg & coconut flour/ almond flour, s&p, pan fry quickly in coconut oil or butter, top with sour cream, and hot sauce.

- **ASPARAGUS**: Toss 1 lb. asparagus with s&p, ⅓ cup parmesan cheese. Spread on parchment lined baking sheet. Cooked 10 mins. at 425 degrees.

- **Mash cauliflower:** add blue cheese & chives.

- **Mix** cauliflower florets, heavy cream, monterey jack, parmesan, goat cheese, s&p, bake 30 mins. at 400 degrees.

- **Sauté spinach**: with butter, s&p. Add pecans, top with swiss cheese, and bake at 350 until cheese is melted.

- **Granny Smith Apples:** shredded, makes a great slaw base.

- **Cold green bean salad:** Cook beans, chill immediately. Add purple onion, feta cheese, toasted nuts, garlic, fresh dill, s&p, and oil & vinegar.

- **Stuff your baby peppers:** Make a slit in one side. Scrape out seeds, stuff with feta cheese. Skewer closed. Toast over open flame, slit side up, until skin is blistered.

ENTRÉES

- **Grilled Eggplant Parm**
- **Pizza Pizzazz!**
- **Avocado Relish Flank Steak**
- **Cowboy Chimichurri**
- **Make Your Pot-Roast**
- **Taco Wraps**
- **Tenderloins 'N Toppers**
- **Don't Let Your Meat-Loaf**
- **Let Your Beef Stew**
- **Lemon Chicken**
- **No Shakin' Just Bakin' Chicken**
- **Stick 'N Chicken**
- **A-Chicken-In-Every-Pot Pie**
- **Chick 'N Parm**
- **Chicken Saltimbocca**
- **Chicken Olē-Olē**
- **Herb Rubbed Chicken-On-The-Bone**
- **Pork Chops 'N Applesauce**

- Grilled Pork with Caper Dressing
- Creamy Herbed Pork Chops
- Pass the Pulled Pork, Please!
- Veal Meatballs with "Mato" Sauce
- Awesome Osso Bucco
- Veal Chop with Olive-Caper Dressing
- Garden Herb Lamb Kebabs
- One-Stop-Lamb Chop
- Spinach 'N Lamb Stir Fry
- Basil 'N Mint Snapper
- Mahi 'N Macadamia's
- Salmon Julienne
- Creamy Dilled Salmon
- Very Crabby Cakes
- Grilled Lime Shrimp
- Clams, Mussels & More

Entrées...Excellence in Every Meal

"The only time to eat diet food is while you're waiting for the steak to cook."

Julia Child
American Chef, Author, Television Personality
1912 - 2004

GRILLED EGGPLANT PARM

"Mato" Sauce (pg. 21), requires prior preparation,
(or use of jarred sauce, no sugar added)

1 large eggplant, washed with skin left on
⅓ cup parmesan cheese, grated
grape seed oil to coat
1-½ cups tomato sauce
1 cup whole milk mozzarella cheese, shredded
sea salt and freshly ground black pepper

Preheat grill to medium
AND
Preheat oven to 400 degrees

Slice eggplant crosswise in ½" thick slices. Sprinkle salt on both sides of eggplant, and stack them (with paper towel in between slices). Place a weight on top of the eggplant (i.e. a heavy pot), and allow the slices to drain for half an hour. Pat dry, and coat both sides of eggplant with grape seed oil. Sprinkle a little more salt and pepper to both sides of the eggplant. Grill for a few minutes on each side. Do not cook until soft, only until grill lines are present. This happens quickly. Remove eggplant and place in a greased (with grape seed oil) large glass baking dish, or dishes. Sprinkle with parmesan cheese. Place two dollops of tomato sauce on each slice to cover completely. Sprinkle with mozzarella cheese. Bake 10 minutes, or until cheese is melted.

There's no harm in parm.

A.W.E. – *cut eggplant thinly, lengthwise.*
Make eggplant rolletini by ADDING ricotta cheese.
Season ricotta with a little red sauce, basil, oregano, sea salt, and pepper.
Stuff and roll eggplant slices
Cover with sauce, and cheese. Heat at 400 degrees for 10 to 12 minutes.

FACT: *Eggplant, is a member of the family of nightshade vegetables.*
Nightshade vegetables may worsen the symptoms of arthritis.
Eggplants are 95% water. Salting an eggplant helps reduce its water content, as well as its bitterness.

PIZZA PIZZAZZ!

**required- pizza stone with a pizza peel
(big wooden pizza spatula)
**required- parchment paper cut to fit pizza stone

For the crust:
1-¼ cups almond flour
3 Tbsps. coconut flour
3 Tbsps. chickpea flour
½ tsp. sea salt
1 tsp. guar gum (pg. 220)
2 eggs
1 egg white
1-½ Tbsps. butter, melted
2 tsps. water

*note: this recipe yields enough dough to make one 10" to 11" pizza

Also required, toppings of your choice such as:
Tomato sauce, mozzarella cheese, pepperoni, meatball, onion,
peppers, olives, mushrooms, etc.

Cut parchment paper to fit pizza stone. Remove parchment paper, and place pizza stone in center rack of oven. Heat to 400 degrees. Place parchment paper on pizza peel (wooden spatula). In a large bowl sift together almond flour, chickpea flour, salt, and guar gum. In a small bowl whisk eggs until frothy, and set aside. Add butter and water to flour mixture. Mix until crumbly, then add the eggs. Form dough into a ball, leaving it in the bowl. Cover with a damp paper towel. Allow to rest for five minutes, then knead dough once again. Form it back into a ball, cover, and let it rest for an additional five minutes. Place dough ball onto the parchment paper on the peel. Place a second piece of parchment on top of the dough and press down into a larger circle. Using a rolling pin (or a flat sided bottle), roll dough to outer edge of cut parchment. Make your pizza dough as thin as desired. Peel off the top piece of parchment, and crimp and roll the outer edge of your dough to form a lip at the edge of the pizza, leaving a ½" or parchment paper around the entire pie. Using the peel, slide your parchment-backed crust onto the heated stone and cook for ten minutes. Using the peel, remove the crust from the oven, leaving the hot stone behind. Remove the parchment paper from the crust, leaving the pizza resting directly on the peel. Add your sauce and toppings of choice. Place your pizza back on the hot stone and cook 7 to 10 minutes, or until cheese is hot and bubbly.

You can keep this dough in the fridge for a day or two,
or freeze it for up to 3 months.

Kiss the cook.

A.W.E. – *OMIT red sauce, ADD pesto with pine nuts,*
and cubed cooked chicken
OR – try using Oh, Dough (pg. 26) as your crust

FACT: *Why use sea salt?*
Table salt is heavily processed,
and may contain a chemical additive to prevent clumping.

Some of the HEALTHIEST, and most NUTRIENT-DENSE veggies are:

Asparagus
Broccoli
Brussels Sprouts
Cauliflower
Collard Greens
Kale
Leek
Lettuce (red & green)
Onions
Peppers
Scallion
Shallot
Spinach

AVOCADO RELISH FLANK STEAK
note: marinate a minimum of 2 hours

1 lb. flank steak, trimmed
2 tsps. fresh lime zest, divided into 2 portions
4 tsps. grape seed oil, divided into 2 portions
1 clove garlic, minced
2 avocados, peeled and diced
½ cup plum tomatoes, chopped
2 Tbsps. red onion, chopped
1 small jalapeño pepper, finely chopped (ribs & seeds removed)
1 Tbsp. fresh lime juice
½ tsp. sea salt, divided into 2 portions
⅛ tsp. freshly ground black pepper

Grill set to medium high heat when marinating is complete

Combine 1 teaspoon of zest, 2 tsps. of grape seed oil, ¼ teaspoon of the salt, pepper and garlic in a small bowl. Score a diamond pattern into both sides of steak. Rub the oil mixture onto both sides, cover and refrigerate for at least 2 hours. Cook steak approximately 6 minutes per side (or until desired degree of doneness). Allow meat to rest for 5 minutes before slicing. Combine the remaining lime zest, 2 tsps. of grape seed oil, salt, diced avocado, tomato, red onion, lime juice, and jalapeño pepper in a small bowl. Meat should be cut into thin slices on the diagonal (across the grain). Serve with relish.

Leave room for dessert.

A.W.E. – *before slicing meat, cover with slices of muenster cheese. Place under broiler quickly until cheese is melted completely*

FACT: *Flank steak is tenderized by marinating, and then grilling, or broiling.*

COWBOY CHIMICHURRI
(bone-in rib eye)

*this recipe requires the making of
Churri-Slurry (chimichurri sauce, pg. 16) BEFORE preparation.

4 bone-in rib eye steaks
1 tsp. garlic powder
sea salt and fresh ground black pepper to taste

Season meat on both sides with: garlic powder, salt and pepper. Cover and refrigerate for at least 1 hour.

Preheat grill to medium heat

Grill for 5 minutes per side (**note: use tongs to turn meat on a grill, not a fork. Forks pierce the meat, allowing juices to escape, making it dry.*) Remove meat and allow to REST for 10 minutes before slicing. Top with a little Churri-Slurry (Chimichurri sauce, pg. 16), serving leftover sauce on the side.

In a chimichurri hurry.

A.W.E. – *OMIT rib eye, and USE Bone, Hanger, Flank,*
Strip steaks, or Ground beef

FACT: *Proteins (amino acids), are an essential part*
of your daily food consumption. Protein defends against illness, and is responsible for muscle repair, tissue growth, hormone regulation, and metabolism control. Our organs, skin, hair, bone, nails, teeth, ligaments, tendons, and muscles are all protein.

MAKE YOUR POT-ROAST

1 (4 lb.) chuck or rump roast
3 tsps. sea salt
2-¾ cups beef stock
1 small onion, chopped
1 tsp. dried thyme
1 tsp. dried ground marjoram
1 bay leaf
3 Tbsps. xylitol sweetener
1 tsp. freshly ground black pepper
4 stalks of celery, chopped
3 medium onions, quartered
3 Tbsps. chickpea flour
2 Tbsps. grape seed oil & 2 Tbsps. coconut oil

Add grape seed and coconut oils to a large pot (with a cover), heat to medium. Trim off any excess fat from roast and salt all sides, using 2 tsps. of salt. Once oil has heated, brown meat on all sides (this takes about 25 minutes). Once browned, add beef stock, 1 small chopped onion, thyme, marjoram, bay leaf, xylitol, pepper, and remaining teaspoon of salt. Cover and reduce heat to low, simmering for 1-½ hours (turn occasionally). Add the celery and three medium onions, re-cover and simmer for an additional 1-½ hours. Remove roast to carving board and allow to rest. Turn pot with liquid back to medium heat. In a small bowl whisk chickpea flour with ½ cup of hot stock. Add flour/broth mixture to pot, stirring well. Remove from heat. Slice your meat, layering it on top of vegetable platter. Garnish with a little gravy.

Just kidding...don't let your pot roast.

A.W.E. – *OMIT bay leaf and marjoram, and ADD rosemary, sage, and thyme*
OR – OMIT roast and ADD a quartered chicken
OR – ADD baby portobello mushrooms

FACT: *The benefits of coconut oil are attributed to the presence of lauric acid, capric acid, and caprylic acid. Coconut oil is soothing, and has anti-microbial, anti-oxidant, anti-fungal, and anti-bacterial properties.*

TACO WRAPS

1 Tbsp. grape seed oil
1 spanish onion, diced
1 green pepper, diced
2-½ lbs. ground beef
1 tsp. chili powder
1 tsp. fresh garlic, chopped
1 tsp. white pepper
1 tsp. chipotle powder
1 can diced tomatoes (or 12 fresh plum tomatoes diced)
1 bunch fresh cilantro, chopped
sea salt to personal taste
boston leaf lettuce, leaves (as taco shell)
*taco toppings of your choice:
sour cream, black or green olives, shredded mexican or
sharp cheddar cheese, diced jalapeño peppers,
cubed tomatoes, shredded iceberg lettuce*

Add grape seed oil to a large sauté pan over medium heat. Cook onion and peppers until half cooked, then add ground beef and all ingredients (except cilantro and boston leaf lettuce). Continue cooking until beef is thoroughly done, stirring occasionally. Remove from heat, add cilantro. Using boston lettuce leaves as taco shells, spoon seasoned beef inside, adding toppings of your choice. Roll up your taco and enjoy. Serve immediately.

No one can eat just one.

A.W.E. – *OMIT ground beef and ADD ground turkey,
OR – chicken pieces OR – shrimp*

FACT: *Proteins cannot be stored for later use
like fat or carbohydrates can, so our bodies need replenishment daily.
Without sufficient protein, our bodies either let cells die,
or break down other muscles and tissues,
to get the protein they need for body repair and other functions.*

TENDERLOINS 'N TOPPERS

4 beef tenderloins
1 large fresh garlic clove, peeled, cut in half
½ tsp. sea salt
optional garnish: 2 tsps. fresh parsley, chopped

TOPPING:
4 tsps. blue cheese, crumbled, room temperature
4 tsps. sour cream
2 Tbsps. cream cheese, softened
2 tsps. yellow onion, minced
White pepper to taste

Preheat oven to broil

In a small bowl combine all topping ingredients, and set aside. Rub both sides of beef with the cut sides of the garlic clove halves. Place tenderloins on broiler rack. Make sure that meat sits 2 to 3 inches from heat. Broil 6 to 8 minutes per side (for medium). Once turned, with 2 minutes remaining, top evenly with blue cheese mixture, and finish cooking. *Cook less for rare to medium rare.* Remove meat. Season immediately with salt, and parsley. Allow meat to rest 10 minutes before serving.

Top that!

A.W.E. – *wrap your beef tenderloins in half-cooked bacon before broiling*

FACT: *¼ cup of fresh parsley provides ⅓ of our daily
vitamin C requirements.
It ranks higher than most vegetables in histidine's
(an amino acid that inhibits tumors).*

DON'T LET YOUR MEAT-LOAF

1-½ lbs. of ground beef (or any combo of veal, pork, or beef)
1 vidalia onion, diced
3 Tbsps. butter
1 cup of pork rinds, coarsely crushed, (pg. 28)
2 eggs
3 Tbsps. prepared horseradish
1 Tbsp. garlic powder
sea salt and freshly ground black pepper
1 Tbsp. bacon fat

Preheat oven to 375 degrees

In a small pan, melt butter and sauté onion until opaque. In a large bowl, mix ground beef with all remaining ingredients. Add the cooked onions and mix well. Place mixture into a greased (with bacon fat), 9" x 13" glass baking dish, forming it into a loaf. Bake uncovered for 35 to 40 minutes, allowing meat to stand for 5 minutes before slicing.

Sit back and enjoy.

A.W.E. *– for a Mexican flavor, OMIT the horseradish,*
and ADD cubed tomatoes, cilantro, and black olives.
Top with shredded cheese before baking,
and serve with a dollop of sour cream.
Taco's without the shell.
OR – top with strips of half-cooked bacon before baking
OR – OMIT horseradish, and ADD 1 Tbsp. each parsley, basil,
oregano, 2 Tbsps. mustard, and ½ cup ketchup

FACT: *Horseradish is high in vitamin C.*
When attempting to make your own horseradish sauce,
do diligent research.
Wear gloves and eye protection.
It is suggested to prepare the root, outdoors if possible.

LET YOUR BEEF STEW

4 lbs. stew beef, cut to 1" cubes
2 Tbsps. coconut flour
2 Tbsps. grape seed
2 Tbsps. butter
4 large onions, sliced
6 cloves garlic, minced
3 Tbsps. xylitol sweetener
6 stalks celery, medium dice
1 tsp. each: onion powder and garlic powder
3 bay leaves
1 Tbsp. each: parsley, thyme, freshly ground black pepper
2 Tbsps. sea salt (plus extra to season beef cubes)
6 cups beef stock
1 head cauliflower (or broccoli) florets, chopped bite-size
2 cups green beans, chopped bite-size
1 zucchini, chopped bite-size

Sprinkle beef cubes with salt and pepper. Dredge in coconut flour. In a large covered pot, sauté the beef cubes in grape seed oil and butter over medium high heat for 5 minutes. Add onions, cooking until beef browns (about 5 minutes), adding garlic when two minutes remain (you don't want it to burn). Reduce heat to low (simmer), and add: xylitol, 3 of the 6 celery stalks, onion powder, garlic powder, bay leaves, parsley, thyme, pepper, salt, and cover all with stock. Cover and cook 90 minutes, stirring occasionally. Add cauliflower, 3 remaining stalks of celery, and cauliflower/broccoli. Cook an additional 30 minutes. Add zucchini, 20 minutes before serving. Season with additional salt and pepper as needed.

Leave room for seconds.

A.W.E. – *OMIT thyme, and ADD cilantro, chili powder,
and a diced red or orange bell pepper*

FACT: *Beef is the third most widely consumed meat in the world (about 25% of meat production worldwide, after pork (38%), and poultry (30%).*

LEMON CHICKEN

8 boneless breast halves
6 eggs
¼ cup lemon juice
½ cup butter
sea salt and freshly ground black pepper
1-½ tsps. fresh garlic, mashed, finely minced
2 Tbsps. chicken stock
¼ cup fresh parsley, finely chopped

Lightly pound chicken breasts to even thickness, between two pieces of parchment paper. In a medium bowl combine eggs and lemon juice, with a little salt and pepper. Melt butter in a large skillet over medium-high heat. Dip the chicken breasts into the egg mixture, and immediately place into the hot pan. Add a little more salt and pepper to taste. Cook 5 to 7 minutes until brown, and turn chicken over. Add garlic to pan, and slowly add chicken stock. Cook an additional 5 to 7 minutes until browned, and no pink remains inside cutlets. Add parsley when done. Serve immediately.

Pass the platter.

A.W.E. – *dust chicken in a combination of ¼ cup almond flour and ¼ cup coconut flour, prior to egg dredge*

FACT: *The lemon tree, is a small evergreen, native to Asia. The juice, pulp, and zest of this brightly colored yellow fruit, are all used in cooking.*

NO SHAKIN', *just* BAKIN' CHICKEN

4 chicken breasts, boneless, skinless

Seasoning:
1 cup pork rinds, finely crushed, seasoned to taste (pg. 28)
¼ cup almond flour
¼ cup coconut flour
½ tsp. guar gum (pg. 220)
2 tsps. celery salt
2 tsps. onion powder
2 tsps. poultry seasoning
1 tsp. paprika
1 tsp. garlic powder
½ tsp. cayenne
½ tsp. sea salt
½ tsp. freshly ground black pepper
(store in an airtight container for a few months)

Wet:
½ cup buttermilk
1 egg, beaten

Preheat oven to 375 degrees

Wash and pat dry chicken, set aside. In a medium size bowl, mix all ingredients for seasoning. Place seasoning in the bottom of a shallow rimmed dish. Mix wet ingredients in a second shallow rimmed dish. One at a time, dip chicken pieces into egg/buttermilk mixture, coating both sides. Allow excess liquid to drip off, and then place cutlet into seasoning, coating both sides. Place seasoned breast on a plate. Repeat steps until all chicken has been coated. Allow to dry before baking. In a glass baking dish, (greased with grape seed oil), cook 30 to 35 minutes, or until no pink remains.

Go back for seconds.

A.W.E. – *OMIT chicken breasts and ADD turkey breasts*

FACT: *Replacement for buttermilk: 1 Tbsp. vinegar or lemon juice and enough milk to equal 1 cup. Allow to stand for 10 mins. before adding to recipe.*

CHICK 'N PARM

*note: "Mato" Sauce (pg. 21) requires prior preparation
(or use of jarred sauce, no sugar added)*

4 chicken breasts, thick-cut, boneless, skinless
8 eggs
sea salt & freshly ground black pepper
2 Tbsps. whole milk
6 cups pork rinds, finely ground and seasoned (pg. 28)
italian seasoning (or herbs of choice)
2 cups tomato sauce
2 cups mozzarella cheese, shredded
½ cup pecorino romano cheese, grated
grape seed oil for frying

Preheat oven to 400 degrees

Pour seasoned crumbs into a dish large enough to hold a chicken breast flat. In a second bowl of the same size, whisk eggs with milk, salt, and pepper. Set both bowls aside. Grease glass baking dishes with grape seed oil. In a large frying pan, add ½" of grape seed oil and bring pan to heat over medium high temperature. Halve chicken breasts (making 8 cutlets). One at a time, place cutlets into egg mixture, then into crumbs, back into egg mixture, and then a second time into crumbs, until each is thoroughly coated. Place immediately into heated pan. Flipping once, cook chicken until no pink remains. Place cooked cutlets into your greased dishes. Sprinkle tops with pecorino-romano cheese, and then top each cutlet with ¼ cup tomato sauce. Lastly, cover cutlets with mozzarella cheese. Bake 10 minutes, or until cheese is completely melted.

No harm, in more parm.

A.W.E. – *cut chicken into smaller pieces to make FINGERS*

FACT: *If you need to make medium-size crushed pork rinds, our "breadcrumbs," use a zip-top bag and a rolling pin. Use light force, so the bag won't fail.*

STICK 'N CHICKEN

4 chicken breasts, boneless, skinless
sea salt and freshly ground black pepper
2 Tbsps. grape seed oil
2 Tbsps. garlic, minced (more to personal taste)
2 bags fresh organic spinach
12 slices fontina cheese, thin
8 large wooden skewers (sticks!)
2 to 3 medium-size shallots, finely chopped
¾ cup chicken broth
2 Tbsps. butter
**oven-friendly skillet

Preheat oven to 350 degrees

Cut chicken breasts in half lengthwise to make cutlets half as thick. Pound breasts out gently for uniformity of thickness. Season both sides of cutlets with salt, and pepper. Add oil to pan and sauté garlic and spinach, until spinach is just wilted. Set aside to cool. Place a heaping spoon of spinach mixture on each chicken cutlet. Lay one and a half slices of fontina cheese on top of the spinach. Carefully roll the breasts tightly from one end to the other. Secure chicken with wooden skewers or large toothpicks. Place chicken in an oven-friendly skillet over med-high heat (seam side down to seal), cooking to light brown on all sides. Add half of the chopped shallots, and sauté quickly (about a minute). Add the chicken broth. Scrape down sides of pan, and place chicken in oven, cooking for 10 minutes. Remove skillet. Place chicken onto a serving tray, and return empty skillet to stovetop. Deglaze pan further by adding rest of shallots, with additional salt and pepper. If too thick, additional broth may be added, but don't over-thin it. Throw butter in at end to finish the sauce. Drizzle over plated chicken and serve.

Stick it, and lick it.

A.W.E. – *ADD crushed red pepper*
OR – *ADD mushrooms*

FACT: *Shallots are known as "multiplier onions,"*
because they are formed in clusters with multiple cloves.
Store shallots in a dry,
dark, cool place, and they can last up to 2 months.
Larger shallots taste more like garlic,
where smaller ones have a sweeter taste.

The CLEAN FIFTEEN

The lowest pesticide contamination resides in these fruits & veggies
(buying organic is not necessary)

Asparagus
Avocado
Broccoli
Cabbage
Eggplant
Kiwi*
Mango*
Onions
Papaya*
Pineapple*
Sweet Corn*
Sweet Peas*
Sweet Potato*
Tomato
Watermelon*

*A low-glycemic eating plan would NOT include
these fruits or veggies

A CHICKEN IN-EVERY-POT PIE

**this recipe requires making ½ recipe for Dough (pg. 26)
prior to assembly.*

2 to 2-½ boneless chicken breasts, cut into bite-size pieces
sea salt
2 cups chicken stock
1 spring fresh rosemary
4 Tbsps. butter
1 medium onion, chopped
1 cup broccoli, chopped
1 cup cauliflower, chopped
1 cup string beans, chopped
½ red bell pepper, chopped
½ green bell pepper, chopped
4 cloves fresh garlic, minced
2 Tbsps. chickpea flour
2 Tbsps. dried parsley
1 tsp. ground sage
additional sea salt
freshly ground black pepper
1 cup cheddar cheese
½ cup heavy cream

Preheat oven to 350 degrees

Grease a deep glass baking dish (with grape seed oil). Salt the pieces of chicken. In a small pot over medium-high heat place stock and fresh rosemary. Once heated, add chicken and cook about 10 minutes, *or until no pink remains inside the largest chicken piece.* Remove rosemary and chicken, but reserve the stock. In a large saucepan melt butter. Add onion, broccoli, cauliflower, green beans, salt and pepper, cooking 5 minutes over medium heat. Add green peppers, red peppers, minced garlic, parsley, sage, garlic, and additional salt and pepper to taste. Mix chickpea flour in some chicken stock until dissolved, then add to pan. Cook an additional five minutes stirring frequently. Add cooked chicken back to pan, stirring well until heated. Transfer to your greased backing dish and sprinkle with cheddar cheese.

Drizzle heavy cream over top. Roll out your prepared crust and cover baking dish. Crimp the edges against the glass, and using a knife, make a few vent holes in the top of the dough. Bake 30 minutes at 350 degrees, then reduce to 325 degrees for an additional 15 minutes. Allow to rest 15 minutes before serving.

Like Mom used to make.

A.W.E. – *OMIT cheddar cheese and ADD swiss or harvarti cheese*

FACT: *Red bell peppers have 2x the amount of Vitamin C (by weight), than citrus fruit.*

There are FIVE SPICES
that may help heal your digestive system

Black Pepper
Cardamom
Coriander
Cumin
Turmeric

We recommend a discussion with your holistic healer regarding the use of these spices, in the specific treatment of any and all illnesses or dysfunction.

CHICKEN SALTIMBOCCA

4 chicken breasts, skinless, boneless, pounded to ¼" thick
1-½ tsps. dried sage
½ tsp. freshly ground black pepper
4 slices prosciutto, thinly sliced
4 Tbsps. butter, melted
2 large bags of pork rinds, finely crushed (pg. 28)
2 Tbsps. parmesan cheese
2 Tbsps. fresh parsley, chopped
8 toothpicks

Preheat oven to 350 degrees

Pound chicken breasts thin, between two pieces of parchment paper. Remove top piece of parchment, and sprinkle sage and pepper over chicken breasts. Place a slice of prosciutto on top. Roll up chicken breasts and prosciutto, removing parchment as you go. Secure chicken with toothpicks. In a shallow dish pour melted butter. In a second dish place the pork rinds, parmesan cheese and parsley, mixing them well. Dip and roll chicken breasts in melted butter and then into the pork rind mixture. Make sure to cover entire cutlet. Place chicken in a greased (with grape seed oil) large glass baking dish (10" x 14"). Bake for 35 to 40 minutes, or until no pink remains. Remove toothpicks before serving.

No licking the plate.

A.W.E. – *top with steamed broccoli,*
and sliced mozzarella cheese (placing under broiler)

FACT: *There are more chickens on earth than there are people,*
over 3 billion in China alone.

CHICKEN OLÉ-OLÉ

4 lbs. chicken legs and thighs (family/value pack)
2 large cans tomatoes, crushed (16 oz.)
4 garlic cloves, skin off, smashed
3 Tbsps. reciato sauce (cilantro puree)
[usually found in the international section of food stores]
1 cup of green manzanilla olives with pimento, drained (sliced or whole)
2 spanish onions, sliced
1 bell pepper (any color), sliced
grape seed oil

Wash chicken and pat dry. In a skillet, place enough grape seed oil to cover pan bottom, and brown chicken. Do NOT cook it through. This is just to add color to the outside of the skin. Place browned chicken into slow cooker or dutch oven. Using the same skillet, sauté the onions, and pepper until onions are just soft. Add sautéed onions, pepper, olives, crushed tomatoes, garlic, and reciato sauce to a slow cooker or large covered pot, set to lowest setting. Cover and cook for 7 hours.

A great day for OLÉ!

A.W.E. – *ADD asparagus*
OR – ADD mushrooms
OR – ADD green beans
OR – OMIT green olives and ADD black olives, or capers

FACT: *Cilantro has anti-inflammatory, as well as strong anti-oxidant properties. It helps promote liver function and is a great source of iron and magnesium.*

HERB RUBBED CHICKEN ON-THE-BONE

4 lbs. (family/value pack) chicken quarters (not separated)
1 cup grape seed oil
2 tsps. garlic powder
2 tsps. sea salt
2 tsps. fresh flat leaf parsley, minced
2 tsps. fresh chives, minced
2 tsps. freshly ground black pepper
2 tsps. fresh rosemary, minced
1 tsp. fresh sage, minced
1 tsp. fresh tarragon, minced

Preheat oven to 350 degrees

Wash and pat dry chicken pieces, loosening the skin from the meat, but do not remove it. Set chicken aside. In a bowl, combine ALL ingredients (except for chicken). Mix well. Lifting the loosened skin of the chicken, place a generous amount of the seasoned oil mixture, under the skin by hand. Apply remaining oil to outside of skin. *Remember to constantly stir oil mixture before applying.* Place chicken directly into a large glass baking dish (you must use a dish with sides). Bake uncovered for 30 minutes. Remove excess oil from the bottom of the pan. Allow the chicken to continue cooking for an additional 30 minutes. This will assure that your chicken stays crispy. Total cooking time will be one hour.

Go ahead...get under their skin.

A.W.E. – *OMIT sage and ADD basil*

FACT: *Sage is known to strengthen memory.*
It is a very good source of vitamins A & K, B6, folate, calcium,
iron, magnesium and manganese.

PORK CHOPS 'N APPLESAUCE

*this recipe requires Granny's Applesauce (pg. 24) be made BEFORE preparation.

4 center cut pork chops (boneless), thinly sliced
2 large bags of pork rinds, crushed medium-fine (pg. 28)
1 tsp. dried sage
1 tsp. dried thyme
1 tsp. dried marjoram OR oregano
sea salt and freshly ground black pepper
3 eggs, whisked
applesauce
grape seed oil

In a lipped, flat dish, pour 2 cups of crushed pork rinds. To the rinds add sage, thyme, marjoram, salt, and pepper, stirring well. Whisk eggs with some salt and pepper, placing mixture in a second lipped dish. Fill a frying pan with approximately ½" of grape seed oil. Set to medium high (about 350 degrees), allowing oil to heat. Take thinly sliced chops, and place into pork rind mixture, lightly coating both sides. Place coated chop into bowl with egg, coating both sides. Place egg covered chop back into pork rinds, and re-coat with seasoned rinds. Carefully place chop into heated oil and proceed to do the same thing to each subsequent chop. Cook approximately 4 to 5 minutes or until a good crunch appears on the bottom but do not allow to burn. Flip chops once, and continue cooking about 3 to 4 more minutes or until no pink remains inside. Remove from oil and place on a dry paper towel to drain. Transfer to serving plate or platter. Serve hot topped with homemade apple sauce.

Just bustin' your chops.

A.W.E. – *for a spicier version, USE spicy pork rinds, and ADD a dash of hot sauce to the whisked eggs*

FACT: *The darker an egg yolk, the more nutritious it is.*

GRILLED PORK
with Caper Dressing

2 (1 lb.) pork tenderloins, trimmed and cut into ¾" slices
3 green tomatoes
¼ cup flat-leaf parsley
3 Tbsps. fresh chives
2 Tbsps. lemon juice
2 Tbsps. grape seed oil
1 Tbsp. capers
1 tsp. fresh oregano
1 tsp. fresh thyme
1 tsp. xylitol sweetener
1 clove garlic
½ tsp. sea salt
1 Tbsp. butter, melted

Preheat grill to medium-high heat

Place slices of tenderloin between two pieces of parchment paper, pounding to ½" thickness. In a food processor, place tomatoes, parsley, chives, lemon juice, grape seed oil, capers, oregano, thyme, xylitol, garlic, and half of the salt, and pepper. Pulse until chunky, or until desired consistency of dressing is achieved. Place mixture to the side. Coat both sides of cutlets with melted butter, and remaining salt & pepper. Place on grill for approximately 5 minutes per side, or until internal temperature reaches 160 degrees. Remove pork, allow to rest. Top with caper dressing.

Clean − your − fork pork.

A.W.E. *– buy the pork as a roast. Make cut marks and insert crushed garlic.*
Oven roast until done using a meat thermometer.
Allow to stand 10 minutes.
Slice and serve with caper dressing.

FACT: *Capers are immature flower buds that are hand harvested.*
The smaller the caper, the more they cost.

CREAMY HERBED PORK CHOPS

4 center cut pork chops, boneless (¾" thick)
sea salt and freshly ground black pepper
1 Tbsp. butter
1 Tbsp. fresh parsley, chopped
1 tsp. coconut flour
1 tsp. chickpea flour
½ tsp. dried basil *OR* tarragon *OR* thyme (crushed)
⅓ cup beef stock
½ cup of heavy cream
2 Tbsps. water
additional fresh parsley, chopped (as garnish)

Sprinkle chops with salt and pepper on both sides. In a large skillet cook chops in butter over medium heat for 5 minutes. Turn chops and cook for an additional 5 to 7 minutes, or until no pink remains. Remove chops, and reserve drippings in pan.

Sauce:

Into the drippings in pan, add the parsley, coconut and chickpea flours, basil (thyme, or tarragon), beef stock, and additional salt and pepper to taste. Mix well and add heavy cream all at once. Cook and stir continuously until thick and bubbly. Stir in water. Return the cooked chops to skillet and heat through, turning once. Remove chops and top with all of the sauce from pan. Garnish with parsley. Serve immediately.

Over — the — top chop.

A.W.E. – *for sauce OMIT ½ tsp. of herb and ADD 1 tsp. of curry and a skinned, cored, finely sliced granny smith apple OR – for a cheesy choice follow same recipe, but ADD ¼ cup of shredded sharp cheddar (or swiss) cheese to sauce after it has thickened*

FACT: *It takes 21 lbs. of whole milk to make 1 lb. of butter.*

PASS THE PULLED PORK, PLEASE

*note: this recipe requires overnight marinating
and use of a slow-cooker*

8 to 9 lb. pork shoulder, boston butt
3 Tbsps. chili powder
3 Tbsps. sea salt
3 Tbsps. freshly ground black pepper
2- 24oz. jars of marinara sauce (no sugar added)
½ cup xylitol sweetener
¾ cup granulated coconut nectar (pg. 220)
¾ cup Faux Brown Sugar (pg. 23)
4 medium yellow onions, quartered
6 cloves fresh garlic, chopped
6 Tbsps. dijon mustard
1-½ cups white vinegar
** Side Suggestion: Summer Slaw (pg. 136),
Requires prior preparation
(Alternate BBQ sauces for cooked pork, pgs. 19 & 20)

Do NOT trim fat off of the boston butt. Combine chili powder, salt, and pepper, then liberally coat the outside of the pork. Cover with plastic wrap and refrigerate overnight. Unwrap and place meat in a slow cooker and cover with garlic and onion pieces. In a large mixing bowl, combine marinara sauce, xylitol, coconut nectar, Faux Brown Sugar, mustard and vinegar. Pour mixture over pork, onions and garlic. Add enough water (or beef stock) to cover pork, until slow cooker is ¾ full. Set on low heat and cook 10 hours, or until meat falls of the bone. Remove meat to cutting board, strain solids from remaining sauce. Using two forks, "shred" the pork and place it back into the bbq sauce until ready to eat. Serve with coleslaw. *Don't forget to freeze your leftovers!*

Need a bib?

A.W.E. – *OMIT pork and ADD two roasting chickens, quartered*

FACT: *Pork is an extremely nutrient dense food,
and one of the highest in thiamin.*

VEAL MEATBALLS with "MATO" SAUCE

*this recipe requires using "MATO" Sauce (pg. 21),
(or use of jarred sauce, no sugar added)

Meatballs:
2 lbs. ground veal
1 cup pork rinds, coarsely crushed (pg. 28)
½ cup parmesan cheese, grated
2 cloves garlic, minced
1-½ tsps. freshly ground black pepper
1 medium yellow onion, minced
1 tsp. dried basil
2 eggs, slightly beaten
¼ cup fresh flat leaf parsley, minced
1 tsp. dried oregano
1 Tbsp. sea salt
¼ cup whole milk
4 Tbsps. butter

In a large bowl, soak pork rinds in milk. After a few minutes, combine all other ingredients except for butter. Mix well. Shape into small meatballs. In a large frying pan over medium heat, melt butter, and add meatballs. Cook until browned. Drain on paper towel. Reheat meatballs in sauce before serving.

Good things come in small packages.

A.W.E. – *OMIT basil and oregano, and ADD capers*

FACT: *Veal is raised on a "milk-based" diet,*
not a grain-fed diet.
It is a good source of B6, B12, and zinc.

VEAL CHOP
with OLIVE-CAPER DRESSING

4 veal chops (1 to 1-¼" thick)
1 Tbsp. dijon mustard
1 Tbsp. fresh lemon thyme, chopped
sea salt and freshly ground black pepper
2 Tbsps. grape seed oil

Dressing
½ cup olive oil
1 clove fresh garlic, peeled
3 anchovy filets
¾ cup pork rinds, whole (not crushed)
⅓ cup fresh parsley
2 Tbsps. capers
1 tsp. lemon zest (rind), grated
1 Tbsp. lemon juice
¼ cup green olives, chopped
sea salt and freshly ground black pepper

Preheat oven to 450 degrees after marinating meat

Cover chops with mustard, lemon thyme, salt and pepper. Place in a zip-top bag, and marinate for 1 hour. In a large oven-friendly skillet, over medium-high heat, add grape seed oil. Sear chops for 2 minutes per side and transfer to oven. Allow to cook 10 to 12 minutes or until chops are just pink inside. Combine olive oil, garlic, anchovies, pork rinds, parsley, capers, and lemon zest in a food processor/ blender. Process ingredients until finely chopped. Add lemon juice, pulsing until just combined. Remove dressing to bowl and add chopped olives, salt, and pepper to taste. Mix well. Serve chops topped with dressing.

Opt...chop.

A.W.E. – *OMIT anchovies, and ADD sun dried tomatoes*
OR – OMIT green olives and ADD black olives

FACT: Thyme has been shown to strengthen the immune system.
Thyme comes in 100 varieties, and is the best known, most widely used herb.
It is sweetest when picked, just as the flower appears.

8 GENETICALLY-ENGINEERED

FOODS TO AVOID

- Canola oil

- Corn

- Cottonseed (used in vegetable oil)

- Crookneck Squash

- Hawaiian Papaya

- Soybeans and Soy Products (including soy sauce manufactured in the U.S.)

- Sugar (from sugar beets)

- Zucchini (some varieties)

AWESOME OSSO BUCCO

*note: "Mato" Sauce (pg. 21) requires prior preparation
(or use of jarred sauce, no sugar added).*

2 lbs. veal shank (cut into rounds through the bone)
2 Tbsps. coconut flour
2 Tbsps. chickpea flour
2 tsps. sea salt
½ tsp. freshly ground black pepper
3 Tbsps. coconut oil
3 Tbsps. butter
1 cup yellow onion, chopped
1 cup celery, chopped
3 cloves garlic, crushed
1 cup tomato sauce
1 cup beef stock
1 tsp. dried basil
4 sprigs fresh thyme, bundled and tied
2 springs fresh rosemary, de-leafed and minced
2 tsps. fresh curly leaf parsley, chopped
1 bay leaf

In a bowl, mix the coconut and chickpea flours with salt and pepper, then dredge veal pieces in flour mixture. On medium heat in a lidded pot, melt butter, and coconut oil. Add veal, browning on all sides. Remove veal and add onion, celery, and garlic, cooking until tender. Add tomato sauce, beef stock, basil, thyme bundle, parsley, rosemary, and bay leaf. Return meat to pot. Bring to boil. Cover and reduce to low, simmering for 3 ½ to 4 ½ hours.

The real deal. Veal.

A.W.E. – *veal cubes (for stew) may be used with, or instead of,
veal shank rounds (for extra meat)*

FACT: *Bay leaf is one of the most widely used culinary herbs.
Its fragrance is much more noticeable than its taste.
Fresh bay leaves are very mild.
Their full flavor is not reached until several weeks after picking and drying.*

GARDEN HERB LAMB KEBABS

1-½ lbs. lamb tenderloin, cut into 2" pieces
2 Tbsps. grape seed oil
3 cloves garlic, minced
¼ cup lemon juice
3 Tbsps. fresh rosemary, chopped
3 Tbsps. fresh mint, chopped
3 Tbsps. fresh thyme, chopped
3 Tbsps. fresh oregano, chopped
2 Tbsps. xylitol sweetener
1 Tbsp. dijon mustard
1 tsp. sea salt
1 tsp. freshly ground black pepper
10 twelve inch skewers
serve on a bed of Citrus Herb Salad (pg. 118)

Preheat grill to medium-high heat after marinating is complete

Combine lamb and all other ingredients into a large zip-top plastic bag, and mix well. Marinate in refrigerator for 30 minutes. Remove lamb and discard marinade. Place lamb onto skewers and grill for 2 minutes on each side. Remove from skewers, and serve over a portion of Citrus Herb Salad.

Whammo ! Lamb, oh !

A.W.E. – *place slices of onion and mushroom*
between cubes of lamb
OR – place tomatoes, and peppers between cubes of lamb

FACT: *Rosemary leaves should almost always be finely chopped,*
unless using an entire sprig.
Rosemary mixes well with chives, parsley, or thyme.

ONE-STOP LAMB CHOP

8 lamb chops
1 garlic clove, minced
½ tsp. dried rosemary
1 tsp. sea salt
½ tsp. onion powder
1 tsp. freshly ground black pepper
2 Tbsps. coconut oil, melted
1 large zip-top bag

Preheat grill to medium heat

Everything...in the bag! Shake well. Allow to sit, room temperature for 10 to15 minutes. Toss chops onto hot grill. Cook about 5 to 7 minutes per side for rare.

Stop 'n chop.

A.W.E. – *OMIT rosemary and ADD parsley*
OR – if don't have a fresh garlic clove handy, use garlic powder

FACT: *Choose heads of garlic that are firm to the touch,*
and that have no nicks or soft cloves.
Fresh garlic is hard to peel.
As cloves age, they shrivel inside of their skins,
and become easier to peel.

SPINACH 'N LAMB STIR FRY

1 lb. boneless leg of lamb (cut into ½" x 2" strips)
1 Tbsp. grape seed oil
2 Tbsps. butter
3 cloves garlic, smashed and minced
6 scallions, diced
2 bell peppers (any color), julienned
1 vidalia onion, julienned
1-¼ cups canned crushed tomatoes
1 tsp. sea salt
1 tsp. ground ginger
1 bag fresh baby spinach

In a large skillet on low heat, melt grape seed oil, and butter. Add garlic, and scallions, cooking until tender. Add bell peppers, and onions, stirring occasionally. Sauté until the onions begin to soften. Raise heat to medium. Add strips of lamb, tomatoes, salt, and ginger. Cook for 5 minutes. Add dry spinach, stirring continuously for 2 minutes. Serve immediately.

Grand slam lamb !

A.W.E. – *if you can't find boneless leg of lamb,*
have the butcher de-bone pork chops, or pork blades
OR – OMIT vidalia onions and ADD pearl onions
OR – ADD mushrooms

FACT: *Lamb is the least favorite red meat*
in North America,
but the favorite meat, in almost every other
country in the world.

BASIL 'N MINT SNAPPER

4 snapper fillets
2 Tbsps. grape seed oil
¼ tsp. sea salt (for fish)
⅛ tsp. freshly ground black pepper

Dressing:
1 cup fresh basil leaves
¼ cup fresh mint leaves
1 jalapeño pepper (seeded)
2 Tbsps. water
2 tsps. fresh lime juice
⅛ tsp. sea salt (for sauce)
1 clove garlic, chopped
olive oil, drizzle (for sauce)
Food processor or blender

Preheat oven broiler

Grease broiler pan (with grape seed oil). Arrange fish in a single layer. Sprinkle with ¼ teaspoon salt, and pepper. Broil the fish for 6 minutes, or until it flakes easily when tested with a fork. While fish cooks, place basil, mint, jalapeño pepper, water, lime juice, ⅛ teaspoon salt, and garlic, into your food processor/blender. Pulse all ingredients, then drizzle (in a continuous stream), enough olive oil to make the sauce smooth. Remove fillets and garnish with sauce. Serve hot.

A "hot" catch.

A.W.E. – *for a less spicy sauce, OMIT jalapeño pepper
and ADD a tomatillo*

FACT: *Mint comes in over 500 varieties.
It is a great compliment to savory, as well as sweet dishes.
Young leaves are much better to use when choosing fresh mint.*

MAHI 'N MACADAMIA'S

4 mahi-mahi fillets (6 oz.)
1 cup almond flour
1 Tbsp. coconut flour
1 Tbsp. chickpea flour
1-½ cups macadamia nuts, coarsely ground
¼ cup butter, melted
sea salt and freshly ground black pepper
2 Tbsps. coconut milk
parchment paper

Preheat oven to 425 degrees

In a medium bowl mix together almond, coconut, and chickpea flours, macadamia nuts, and butter. Set aside. Place a piece of parchment paper in the bottom of a glass baking dish, and lightly grease the paper with grape seed oil. Season both sides of the mahi-mahi with salt and pepper to taste. Place the fillets on the parchment. Bake uncovered for 5 minutes. Remove from oven and brush each fillet with coconut milk. Divide the nut mixture among the tops of all four fillets. Pat mixture down on the tops of fillets, so that it adheres and evenly covers. Return to oven and bake for 4 to 6 minutes, or until fish flakes easily.

Drive your fish nuts!

A.W.E. – *OMIT macadamia nuts and ADD toasted almonds*
OR – ADD a little thai chili paste for great thai flavor

FACT: *Mahi-mahi is commonly known as Dorado fish,*
or Dolphin fish. Many people mistakenly believe that the Dolphin fish,
is the same as the mammal we call Dolphin.
They are two totally different things. Really!
No worries, you are NOT eating 'Flipper.'

SALMON JULIENNE

4 wild salmon fillets
2 zucchini, julienned
2 summer squash, julienned
2 red bell peppers, julienned
2 green bell peppers, julienned
1 stick butter, melted
sea salt and freshly ground black pepper
aluminum foil (4 large squares, one for each fillet)
parchment paper (4 large squares, one for each fillet)

Preheat oven to 350 degrees

Take the four pieces of foil and line them with parchment paper. *Never allow aluminum to come in direct contact with your food.* Place one fish fillet in the center of each piece of parchment. In a large bowl, place all julienned vegetables. Pour butter over veggies, and toss well. Season with salt and pepper to taste. Arrange veggies on the top of each fillet. Using double folds on edges, close and secure parchment-lined foil around fish. Do not pull foil tight. Allow space for steam to build and keep fish moist. Place foil pouches in large glass baking dish, or a pan with low sides. Bake for 25 minutes. Fish will easily flake with a fork when done.

A great fish dish.

A.W.E. – *OMIT salmon and ADD your favorite fish fillets*
OR – OMIT plain butter and ADD an Herb Butter (pg. 28)
OR – place fresh dill and sliced lemon on top of veggies before cooking

FACT: *Although farm raised salmon is available in endless supply,*
wild salmon is much healthier for you.
Wild salmon fillet: have:
10x less the amount of PCB's than farm-raised varieties,
contain less parasites,
and are higher in Omega 3 fatty acids.

CREAMY DILLED SALMON

*this recipe requires parchment paper

Sauce:
⅓ cup mayonnaise (pg. 7)
⅓ cup sour cream
1 Tbsp. onion, finely chopped
1 tsp. prepared horseradish
1 tsp. lemon juice
¼ tsp. garlic salt
1 tsp. dill weed
freshly ground black pepper to taste

Entrée:
2 lbs. salmon fillets
1-½ tsps. lemon pepper seasoning
1 tsp. onion salt
1 small onion, sliced into rings
6 lemon slices
¼ cup butter, cubed

Preheat oven to 350 degrees

Place all ingredients for SAUCE in a bowl, and whisk until smooth. In a large rimmed baking dish (or 2 smaller ones), place a piece of parchment paper (large enough to seal at the top, crimped, over the fish). Place fish skin-side down, and sprinkle with lemon pepper & salt. Top each fillet with an onion ring and a slice of lemon. Place a few pats of butter on each fillet. Fold parchment at the top, and staple closed. Bake 20 minutes. Cut top of parchment off, exposing fish. Set oven to broil. Move fish 4" to 6" from heating element, and cook 8 to 12 minutes, until fish flakes easily.

Oven or grill, fish love dill.

A.W.E. – *OMIT dill and ADD parsley*
OR – *OMIT lemon pepper, lemon juice & lemon slices,
and ADD 2 tsps. Dijon mustard to the sauce*

FACT: *Dill seeds and leaves are great culinary herbs.
It's a member of the parsley family, with light green feathery leaves.
Dill water is given to fussy babies as a digestive aid.*

VERY CRABBY CAKES

note: Dippy Fishy (Tartar Sauce, pg. 10) requires prior preparation

3 lbs. jumbo lump crabmeat
1 Tbsp. fresh lemon juice
6 scallions, finely chopped
¾ cup flat-leaf parsley, finely chopped
1 Tbsp. old bay seasoning
1-½ tsps. dry mustard
3 large eggs
1-½ cups Mayonnaise (pg. 7)
grape seed oil for frying

Preheat oven to 200 degrees

Take the time to inspect crabmeat, making sure to remove all cartilage or pieces of shell. Work carefully to preserve the large lumps of crabmeat. Place crab in large bowl, add lemon juice, scallions, parsley, old bay seasoning, and mustard. Gently fold ingredients in, without breaking up the crab. In a small bowl, beat the eggs, and add the mayonnaise, combining well. Gently fold egg/mayonnaise mixture into the crab meat.

Place crab mixture into a large strainer, set over a bowl and cover with plastic wrap. Allow crab to drain overnight if possible (for several hours at a minimum). Form crab mixture into 12 separate, 3" diameter, ½" thick cakes, (about ½ cup each). Cover, and store in refrigerator until ready to cook. Heat oil in cast iron skillet over medium heat. Place half the crab cakes in pan, and cook for 3 minutes without moving them, or until well browned. Flip and cook for another 3 minutes until second side is browned. Transfer to a glass baking dish. Place them in a warm oven, until remaining cakes are cooked. Serve with Dippy Fishy Tartar Sauce (pg. 10).

A little dabby of crabby.

A.W.E. – *OMIT parsley and ADD cilantro OR dill*
OR – ADD cooked, crumbled bacon and one bell pepper

FACT: *1.5 million tons of crabmeat are consumed worldwide each year. Crabs account for one fifth of ALL creatures caught in ALL bodies of water around the globe.*

GRILLED LIME SHRIMP

2 lbs. large shrimp, peeled & deveined
¼ cup fresh lime juice
2 shallots, minced
2 cloves garlic, minced
sea salt and freshly ground black pepper
½ cup grape seed oil

bamboo skewers (soaked in water for one hour, prior to use)

Preheat grill to medium heat after shrimp have marinated

In a non-metallic bowl combine lime juice, shallots, garlic, salt, and pepper. Slowly add oil, whisking well. Place shrimp in a zip-top bag, and add marinade. Refrigerate from 1 to 3 hours (at the most). Place 3 or 4 shrimp per skewer, making sure to skewer tail and head of each one. Place skewers on heated grill and cook for 1 to 2 minutes per side. Remove shrimp from skewers, and serve immediately.

Don't skimp on the shrimp.

A.W.E. – *ADD sea scallops WITH or INSTEAD of shrimp*
OR – ADD fresh rosemary to the marinade for a different flavor

FACT: *Be extremely aware of the time you allow
shrimp to sit in an acidic marinade.
Acidic marinades begin to cook shrimp prior to exposing
them to a heat source.
Acidic marinades can discolor aluminum dishes, bowls, or pans.*

CLAMS, MUSSELS & MORE

2 lbs. mussels
24 little neck clams
1 lb. cockles
1 stick of butter
4 shallots, chopped
2 garlic cloves, minced
1 pint grape tomatoes
12 fresh basil leaves, julienned
1 can coconut milk (14 oz.)

Wash all seafood shells thoroughly!
Clam shells should all be closed tightly.
Discard any open ones,
including those that are chipped, or damaged.
Remove the "beard" from the mussels (see FACT).

In a large pot, melt butter on low heat. Add shallots and garlic. Sauté for 8 to 10 minutes. Add the tomatoes, mashing against the side of the pot (so they are no longer whole). Add 6 of the basil leaves, and all of the coconut milk. Allow mixture to simmer for 15 minutes. Add the remaining basil leaves, and cleaned shellfish. Stir well. Cover and continue simmering about 30 minutes. Stir occasionally, to get top shells to bottom, and vice-versa. All shells are done when opened. Serve hot.

Show us your mussels !

A.W.E. – *ADD chunks of swordfish or sea scallops*
OR – ADD red curry paste to give it a thai twist

FACT: *The byssal threads of a mussel (the beard) are comprised of many fibers. Giving the beard a sharp "yank" toward the hinged-end will not kill the mussel. Yanking the beard out toward the side that opens, can tear the mussel on the inside of the shell, which kills it. Discard byssal threads once removed.*

More Helpful Hints and Ideas

- **BURGER STUFFERS**: Stuff the center of your burger before cooking. With things like cheese, bacon, BBQ Sauce (pgs. 19 & 20), sautéed onions, or Creamed Spinach (pg. 132).

- **PESTO your burger**: Mix Pesto (pg. 17) into your beef. Top your cooked, pesto-cheeseburger with cheese and Avocado Ranch Dressing (pg. 121).

- **Chicken Idea**: Cover 4 boneless chicken breasts with ½ cup Mayonnaise (pg. 7), ¼ cup parmesan/or romano cheese, and 1 Tbsp. prepared horseradish. Sprinkle seasoned, crushed pork rind breadcrumbs (pg. 28) on top. Bake 425 for 20 minutes.

- **Chicken Rollers**: Pound breasts to ⅛", spread with cream cheese and sweet onion, roll chicken. Wrap with cooked (but not crisp) bacon. Secure with toothpicks. Bake in glass dish at 350 degrees until cooked through (approx. 30 mins.), or until no pink remains.

- Take two **grilled chicken cutlets**, and put cheese, bacon, and your favorite dressing in the middle. A true "chicken sandwich."

- Top your **grilled skirt steak** with gorgonzola cheese.

- **Stuff your whole fish-** with lemon, butter, and your favorite herbs before you grill it.

- **Bake your sausage (just like your bacon)** if you don't want to fry it, or you don't own a grill.

- **Save the meatballs**: To keep meatballs from falling apart when frying, refrigerate them for 30 minutes before cooking.

- **Overdone the garlic?**: If your soup or stew is flavored too heavily with garlic for your taste, try adding a sprig of parsley to the pot and allow it to simmer for ten minutes.

DESSERTS

- **Peanut Butter Fudge Mousse**
- **Chillin' Raspberry Cheesecake**
- **Chocolate Dunkin' Cookies**
- **Lovin' Raspberry Cookies**
- **Eat, Gingerly...Cookies**
- **Peanutty Cookies**
- **Ooorange-Chocolate Dippers**
- **Classic Vanillahhh Cake**
- **Crazy for Coconut Cake**
- **Dad's Great Chocolate Cake**
- **Dad's Greater Chocolate Icing**
- **Lemon-Heaven Bars**
- **Mini-Razzy Cupcakes**

- **Put-De-Lime-In-De-Coconut Cupcakes**
  - **Cravin' Chocolate Cupcakes**
    - **Lime-Time Pie**
      - **Gibbles**
      - **Buddies**
    - **"Faux" Fried Ice Cream**
      - **Whippin' Good**
    - **Creamin' Cheese Icing**
      - **Posh Ganache**
    - **Butter 'N Cream Icing**
      - **Raspberry Glaze**
  - **Orange-Chocolate Drizzle**

Delicious Dessert...Guilt-free

"It is health that is real wealth, and not pieces of gold and silver."

Mahatma Gandhi
Preeminent Leader
of Indian Nationalism in British-ruled India
1869 - 1948

PEANUT BUTTER FUDGE MOUSSE

½ cup + 2 Tbsps. heavy cream
3 Tbsps. butter, softened
½ cup cream cheese, softened
2 tsps. vanilla extract
6 Tbsps. xylitol sweetener, powdered
(in a coffee bean grinder)
¼ cup natural chunky peanut butter, *no sugar added*
2 oz. malitol-sweetened milk chocolate, (pg. 219)

*optional garnish: 2 Tbsps. salted peanuts, chopped,
and Whipped Cream (pg. 212)*

Whip ½ cup of heavy cream into firm peaks. Chill until ready to use. In a separate mixing bowl combine butter, cream cheese, vanilla, and xylitol. Beat ingredients until thick and fluffy. Lastly, add peanut butter. Fold in chilled whipped cream. In a small double boiler, heat the 2 Tbsps. heavy cream, and milk chocolate until chocolate is melted. Stir until completely smooth, and remove from heat. Cool chocolate for about 4 minutes. Fold most of the chocolate into the peanut butter mixture, reserving 2 Tbsps. for garnish. This dessert is very rich, small portions are suggested. Garnish by placing a dollop of whipped cream on top, drizzled with remaining chocolate, and sprinkle a few peanuts on top. Serve immediately.

*Duck, duck, goose.
We want mousse !*

A.W.E. – *OMIT peanut butter and ADD sunflower butter (or any nut butter)
OR – USE creamy peanut butter rather than chunky*

FACT: *It takes 540 peanuts to make 12 oz. of peanut butter.*

CHILLIN' RASPBERRY CHEESECAKE

note: make Toasted Pecan Crust (pg. 27), before cheesecake

24 oz. cream cheese, softened
¾ cup xylitol sweetener, finely ground
(in a coffee grinder)
5 eggs
3 Tbsps. coconut flour
1 tsp. vanilla
¼ cup heavy cream
7 oz. coconut milk (half a can)
7 Tbsps. raspberry jelly,
(fruit-sweetened only, with or without seeds)
crust

Preheat oven to 325 degrees

In a bowl beat cream cheese and add xylitol until well combined. Add eggs, one at a time, until each egg is mixed in, but do not over mix. Add coconut flour, vanilla, heavy cream, coconut milk, and 3 Tbsps. of raspberry jelly, and stir lightly. *If you don't want a crust,* pour directly into a greased (with coconut oil), 9" x 13" glass baking dish. *If you have chosen to make the toasted pecan crust, first you must ladle, don't pour the cheesecake batter, or you will destroy your crust.* In a small bowl, use the back of a spoon to mash the remaining jelly, stirring until runny. Drizzle jelly on top of cake in 2 or 3 lines running the length of the pan. Using a blunt knife, "cut" or "swirl" the jelly into the cheesecake for color. Bake approximately 45 to 50 minutes, or until edges start to brown. Toothpick inserted into cake will come out clean when done. Remove from oven and allow to cool. Cover and refrigerate overnight for best results. Remove cheesecake from refrigerator 30 minutes before serving.

Chillin' 'n fillin'.

A.W.E. – *OMIT coconut milk and ADD 1 cup of sour cream*

FACT: *Coconut milk can replace electrolyte loss from perspiration.*

CHOCOLATE DUNKIN' COOKIES

9 Tbsp. Butter, softened
¾ cup xylitol sweetener, ground finely
(in a coffee bean grinder)
1 egg
½ tsp. vanilla
½ cup + 3 Tbsps. almond flour
¼ cup + 1 Tbsp. coconut flour
1 tsp. guar gum (pg. 220)
½ tsp. baking soda
⅓ cup cocoa powder, unsweetened
2 parchment lined baking sheets

Preheat oven to 350 degrees

In a large bowl mix butter and xylitol. Add egg and vanilla extract. Into wet ingredients SIFT: almond flour, coconut flour, guar gum, baking soda, and cocoa. Mix well. Using dampened hands, form dough into walnut-size pieces. Place dough 2" apart on baking sheets. Bake in SINGLE layer (one cookie sheet at a time), for best results. Bake 14 minutes, or until set. Allow to cool on baking sheet before transferring to wire rack. Cool completely. These set up great, placed in an airtight container in the refrigerator. Separate layers with parchment paper.

Cookie dunkin',
beats doughnut dunkin'.

A.W.E. *– poke a little crater in top of a walnut-size piece of dough*
(using the back of a wet wooden spoon),
and put a dab of peanut butter inside the crater

FACT: *Vanilla is the only edible fruit belonging to the family of orchids.*
Out of 150 varieties, only 2 are used commercially.

LOVIN' RASPBERRY COOKIES

1 cup butter, softened
¾ cup xylitol sweetener, finely ground
(in a coffee bean grinder)
1 egg yolk
1 tsp. raspberry extract
1-½ cups almond flour
½ cup coconut flour
1 tsp. guar gum (pg. 220)
pinch of sea salt
1 cup unsweetened coconut, shredded
4 Tbsps. raspberry jelly (fruit-only sweetened)
2 parchment lined baking sheets

Preheat oven to 375 degrees

In a large bowl, beat butter and xylitol. Add egg yolk and raspberry extract. Into the wet ingredients SIFT: almond flour, coconut flour, guar gum, and salt. Mix well. Add shredded coconut, stirring until combined. Form dough into walnut-size balls and place them 2" apart on parchment-lined baking sheets. *These cookies do spread.* Using the back handle of a wooden spoon (dampened), make a hole in the center of each ball, and fill with raspberry jelly. Bake in a single layer (one baking sheet at a time), for 14 to 16 minutes until golden brown. Cool on baking sheet for 5 minutes, then transfer to wire baking rack to cool completely. Store in an airtight container, refrigerated, with layers separated by parchment paper. Makes two dozen cookies.

Share with a friend

A.W.E. – *OMIT raspberry extract/jelly and ADD
the extract and jelly of your favorite berry*

FACT: *Russia is the number one raspberry producer in the world,
at 95,000 TONS per year.*

EAT, GINGERLY...COOKIES

1-¾ cups almond flour
½ cup coconut flour
¼ cup chickpea flour
1 tsp. baking soda
1-¼ tsps. guar gum (pg. 220)
¾ tsp. ground cinnamon
½ tsp. ground cloves
¼ tsp. sea salt
¾ cup butter, softened
1 cup xylitol sweetener
1 egg
¼ tsp. maple extract
¼ cup Nature's Hollow sugar-free honey
2 tsps. ground ginger
2 Tbsps. xylitol sweetener, (in a small dish)

Preheat oven to 350 degrees

In a large bowl, SIFT: almond flour, coconut flour, chickpea flour, baking soda, guar gum, cinnamon, cloves, ginger, and salt. Set aside. In a separate bowl, cream together butter and 1 cup of xylitol. Beat in egg, maple extract, and sugar-free honey. Combine dry ingredients into wet ingredients mixing well. Form dough into walnut-size balls, and roll in the remaining 2 Tbsps. of xylitol. Place dough onto a parchment-lined cookie sheet, about 3 inches apart. Press down lightly on each ball, in a crisscross pattern (using the back of a fork). Bake approximately 14 minutes, or until edges begin to darken. Transfer soft cookies (along with the parchment), to a cooling rack. Store layered, in an airtight container in the refrigerator. Cookies firm when chilled. Makes two dozen cookies.

Don't forget a cold glass of milk

A.W.E. – *ADD some Cream Cheese Icing (pg. 213)*
OR – Whipped Cream (pg. 212) as a garnish

FACT: *Almond Flour is made from almonds that have had the oil extracted from them, giving it a slightly drier consistency than Almond Meal.*

PEANUTTY COOKIES

9 Tbsps. butter, softened
½ cup chunky peanut butter (no sugar added)
1 cup xylitol sweetener
1 egg
¾ cup almond flour
¼ cup coconut flour
1 tsp. guar gum (pg. 220)
½ tsp. baking powder
pinch sea salt
¾ cup peanuts
2 parchment lined baking sheets

In a large bowl, mix butter and peanut butter. Add xylitol, a little at a time, until combined. Add egg. Into the butters SIFT: almond flour, coconut flour, guar gum, baking powder, and salt. Stir well. Add peanuts. Once combined, form dough into ball, cover, and refrigerate for 30 minutes.

Preheat oven to 375 degrees

Form dough into 24 balls, placing them on baking sheets, 2" apart, flattened slightly. Bake in single layer (one baking sheet at a time), for 17 minutes, or until golden brown. Cool completely. Store layered (with parchment paper), in an airtight container in refrigerator.

Smile in between bites.

A.W.E. – *OMIT peanut butter and peanuts
and ADD almond butter and almonds
OR – cashew butter and cashews*

FACT: *Peanuts are known in many countries, by other names;
earthnuts, goober peas, monkey nuts, pygmy nuts,
ground nuts, and pig nuts.*

OOORANGE-CHOCOLATE DIPPERS

*this recipe requires overnight refrigeration before dipping.

1 cup butter, softened
¼ cup xylitol sweetener, finely ground
(in a coffee bean grinder)
1 Tbsp. orange zest
1 egg yolk
2 tsps. orange extract
1-½ cups almond flour
¼ cup coconut flour
¼ cup chickpea flour
1 tsp. guar gum (pg. 220)
1 tsp. ground ginger
pinch of sea salt
4 oz. malitol-sweetened chocolate bar (pg. 219)
OR unsweetened baker's chocolate sweetened to personal taste
2 parchment lined baking sheets

In a large bowl place butter, xylitol, and orange zest. Combine well. Add egg and orange extract. Into wet ingredients SIFT: almond flour, coconut flour, chickpea flour, guar gum, ginger, and salt, mixing well. Form dough into a large ball, cover and refrigerate 1 hour.

Preheat oven to 375 degrees

Form walnut-size balls and place 1-½" apart on baking sheet. Press cookies flat. Bake in single layers (one sheet at a time), for 14 to 16 minutes, or until golden brown. Chill completely. Cover and refrigerate overnight on baking sheets. Melt chocolate in a double boiler the next day. Dip half the cookie in chocolate, placing it back on the parchment lined baking sheet. Refrigerate until set. Store in airtight container, in layers, separated by parchment paper.

Make a cup of tea...quick!

A.W.E. – *OMIT orange extract and ADD lime extract*

FACT: *Orange zest is popular in cooking because its strong oil glands have a distinct flavor that mimics the fleshy insides of an orange.*

CLASSIC VANILLAHHH CAKE

1 cup xylitol sweetener
¾ cup butter, softened slightly
4 eggs
1 tsp. vanilla
½ cup milk
1-½ cups almond flour
½ cup coconut flour, sifted
1 tsp. guar gum (pg. 220)
2 tsps. baking powder
optional garnish: Whipped Cream (pg.212), and fresh berries

Preheat oven to 350 degrees

Cream together xylitol and butter until smooth. Add eggs one at a time, stirring well between each one. Add vanilla and milk. In a separate bowl, SIFT: almond flour, coconut flour, guar gum, and baking powder. Add dry ingredients, to wet ingredients a little at a time, combining until creamy. Grease (with coconut oil) a 10" x 14" glass baking dish *(for a thicker cake use a 9" x 13" glass dish and bake longer.)* Spread batter into dish, spreading evenly. Bake 24 to 26 minutes, or until edges turn light brown, and toothpick inserted into center of cake comes out clean. Remove from oven and allow to cool completely. Serve with fresh berries and whipped cream.

Everyone loves a classic.

A.W.E. – *pour strawberries (marinated in xylitol, and a little lemon juice),
on top with whipped cream,
for gluten-free strawberry shortcake
OR – drizzle with a little chocolate topping (pgs. 214 & 217)*

FACT: *As butter is essentially milk fat,
it contains only traces of lactose, so moderate consumption of butter
is normally not an issue for people suffering
with lactose intolerance.*

CRAZY for COCONUT CAKE

1 cup coconut milk
1 cup xylitol sweetener
2 eggs
½ tsp. vanilla extract
¼ tsp. coconut extract
¾ cup almond flour, sifted
¼ cup coconut flour, sifted
1 tsp. guar gum (pg. 220)
2 tsps. baking powder
¼ tsp. sea salt
*optional garnish: Whipped Cream (pg. 212)
and toasted coconut*

Preheat oven to 350 degrees

Grease (with coconut oil) a large glass baking dish (10" x 14"). Lightly sprinkle the dish with 1 tsp. of the coconut flour. In a bowl, mix coconut milk, xylitol, eggs, vanilla, and coconut extract. In a separate bowl SIFT: almond flour, coconut flour, guar gum, baking powder, and salt. Stir dry ingredients into wet ingredients, mixing well. Pour batter into baking dish. Bake 35 minutes, or until sides appear a light golden brown. Toothpick inserted into cake should come out clean when done. Remove cake from oven, allowing it to cool completely. Garnish with whipped cream, and toasted coconut.

Cuckoo for coconut.

A.W.E. – *serve with Berry Glaze (pg. 216)*
OR – with fresh raspberries topped with Whipped Cream (pg. 212)

OR – sprinkle toasted coconut on top of cake, hot out of the oven.
Toast coconut on parchment-lined cookie sheet,
4 minutes @ 350 degrees. Sprinkle with sweetener while hot, and mix well.

FACT: *Coconut oil stimulates metabolism,*
increases energy and improves thyroid function.

DAD'S GREAT CHOCOLATE CAKE

2 cups almond flour
½ cup coconut flour
½ cup chickpea flour
½ cup cocoa powder, unsweetened
1 tsp. baking soda
1 tsp. salt
2 tsps. guar gum (pg. 220)
2 cups xylitol sweetener
2 cups hot water
½ cup grape seed oil
2 Tbsps. distilled white vinegar
1 Tbsp. instant decaf coffee granules
1 Tbsp. vanilla extract

Preheat oven to 350 degrees

Into a large bowl, SIFT: almond flour, coconut flour, chickpea flour, cocoa, baking soda, salt, and guar gum. Once combined add xylitol. In a separate bowl combine hot water, grape seed oil, vinegar, coffee, and vanilla. Mix well and add to dry ingredients. Divide batter between two greased (with a grape seed oil) glass pie dishes, or a large 9" x 14" glass baking dish (which will increase cooking time). Using the palm of your hand, push down slightly in center of the batter of both cakes. Bake 26 to 28 minutes, or until toothpick inserted in the center of cake, comes out clean. Cool completely before icing.

DAD'S GREATER CHOCOLATE ICING

1 stick butter
1-½ cups xylitol sweetener
1 tsp. instant decaf coffee granules
1-¼ cups cocoa powder, unsweetened
⅛ tsp. salt
1-¼ cups heavy whipping cream
¼ cup sour cream
2 tsps. vanilla extract

Melt butter in saucepan over medium heat. Add xylitol and coffee, stirring until completely melted. Add cocoa and salt. In a medium size bowl combine heavy cream, and sour cream. Once combined, slowly add to the chocolate mixture, stirring until smooth. Cook approximately 8 to 10 minutes, until hot throughout. Remove from heat and add vanilla. Cool icing to room temperature. Pour icing over top(s) of cake(s). Cover and refrigerate them for a minimum of 6 hours (overnight is best).

With cold milk...or hot tea ?
Decisions. Decisions.

A.W.E. *– make recipe as cupcakes, filling mini-liners about 2/3 full.*
Using the end of a wooden spoon,
Push down the centers of each mini cupcake, leaving a small indentation.
Bake 14 to 16 minutes, or until a toothpick inserted, comes out clean.

OR – OMIT coffee, and ADD fresh raspberries or extract

FACT: *Cocoa (unsweetened) is a good source of protein, potassium, and zinc. It's a very good source of iron, magnesium, phosphorus, copper, and manganese.*

LEMON-HEAVEN BARS

⅓ cup butter, softened
½ cup almond flour
½ cup coconut flour
2 tsps. lemon extract
1 tsp. guar gum (pg. 220)
1 cup xylitol sweetener
2 eggs
2 Tbsps. almond flour
4 Tbsps. lemon juice
¼ tsp. baking powder

Preheat oven to 350 degrees

In a small bowl beat butter for 30 seconds. Add only ¼ cup of xylitol, and mix well. Into butter SIFT: ½ cup almond flour, coconut flour, and guar gum. Add 1 tsp. of lemon extract. Mix well and press into bottom of an 8" x 8" glass baking dish (greased with coconut oil). Bake 10 minutes. *Meanwhile:* In small bowl beat: eggs, lemon juice, remaining ¾ cup xylitol, remaining 1 tsp. of lemon extract, baking powder, and 2 Tbsps. almond flour, for two minutes until smooth. Ladle mixture on top of baked crust, and return to oven. Bake 30 minutes, or until edges are lightly brown. Allow to cool completely before cutting. Refrigerate leftovers.

Lemon smiles.

A.W.E. – *ADD a dab of Cream Cheese Icing (pg. 213)*
(flavored with lemon perhaps)

FACT: *Choose lemons colored a rich, bright yellow,*
with no signs of immature green patches.
Lemons should be large, firm, and heavy for their size.
ZEST from a lemon or lime,
may be stored in an airtight container, in a cool, dry place.

MINI-RAZZY CUPCAKES

1-½ cups raspberries, cut in quarters
(to lessen the "graying" of cupcake batter, leave berries whole)
1 cup xylitol sweetener
8 oz. cream cheese, softened
3 eggs
1 tsp. vanilla extract
¾ cup + 2 Tbsps. almond flour
¼ cup + 2 Tbsps. coconut flour
1 tsp. guar gum (pg. 220)
1 tsp. baking soda
pinch sea salt

**optional garnish: Whipped Cream (pg. 212),
OR Cream Cheese Icing (perhaps raspberry flavored) (pg. 213)*

Preheat oven to 350 degrees

Place paper liners in mini-muffin baking sheets. Combine raspberries with only ¼ cup xylitol, and set aside. In separate bowl, beat cream cheese and remaining xylitol until well mixed. Add one egg at a time, incorporating well after each addition. Stir in vanilla extract. Into wet ingredients SIFT: almond flour, coconut flour, guar gum, baking soda, and salt. Reserving enough sweetened raspberries pieces (1 for each muffin), fold remaining berries into dough. Fill mini-muffin liners with batter, placing one berry piece on top of each. Bake 13 to 15 minutes, or until toothpick comes out clean. Refrigerate in airtight containers.

Don't blow raspberries. Eat them.

A.W.E. – *ADD ½ cup chopped nuts, or some fresh mint leaves, minced*

FACT: *The successful yields in raspberry crops, are credited to the plants ability to self-pollinate. Bees transfer pollen to the same plant they get it from eliminating the need for a male and female plant.*

PUT-DE-LIME-IN-DE-COCONUT CUPCAKES

1 cup almond flour
¼ cup coconut flour
1 tsp. guar gum (pg. 220)
1 tsp. baking powder
pinch of sea salt
¾ cup xylitol sweetener, finely ground
(in a coffee grinder)
2 Tbsps. butter, softened
½ cup whole milk
1 tsp. vanilla extract
¼ tsp. coconut extract
2 eggs
½ cup coconut flakes, unsweetened

For Icing:
8 oz. cream cheese, softened; 2 Tbsps. butter, softened;
2 Tbsps. lime juice; zest of 2 limes; ½ cup heavy cream
6 Tbsps. xylitol sweetener, powdered

Preheat oven to 350 degrees

Batter:

In a medium bowl, SIFT: almond flour, coconut flour, guar gum, baking powder, and salt. In a separate bowl mix xylitol, butter, milk, vanilla and coconut extracts. Add one egg at a time, to the wet ingredients, incorporating well after each addition. Slowly add the dry ingredients to the wet ingredients, mixing well. Add flaked coconut and combine. In a paper-lined muffin baking sheet, fill each muffin paper two thirds of the way up, with batter. Bake for 22 to 24 minutes. Allow to cool completely. Store in airtight container in the refrigerator.

Icing:

Whip the cream cheese, butter, zest, and lime juice. Once combined add xylitol. Mix well. In a separate bowl, whip heavy cream to stiff peaks. Fold whipped cream (in small batches) into the cream cheese mixture. Cover and refrigerate. Ice cupcakes before serving.

Sing for your dessert.

A.W.E. – *OMIT flaked coconut*
OR – sprinkle toasted, shredded coconut on top of icing,
(coconut toasts 4 minutes in a 350 degree oven)

FACT: *One third of the world's population*
depends on coconut
to some degree, for food or economics.

8 FOODS TO BOOST YOUR IMMUNITY

Bioflavonoids
Carotenoids
Garlic
Omega-3 Fatty Acids
Selenium
Vitamin C
Vitamin E
Zinc

We recommend a discussion with your holistic healer
regarding the importance and need for any of these
in the specific treatment of any, and all, illnesses or dysfunction.

CRAVIN' CHOCOLATE CUPCAKES
(with Peanut Butter Filling)

Filling:
3 oz. cream cheese, softened
¼ cup + 1 Tbsp. peanut butter
4 Tbsps. xylitol sweetener
1 Tbsp. heavy cream

Batter:
1 cup water
¼ cup grape seed oil
1 Tbsp. white vinegar
1 tsp. vanilla extract
1-¼ cups almond flour
¼ cup + 2 Tbsps. coconut flour
1-½ tsps. guar gum (pg. 220)
1 cup xylitol sweetener
¼ cup cocoa powder, unsweetened
1 tsp. baking soda
½ tsp. sea salt

Preheat oven to 350 degrees

Filling:

In a large bowl, beat cream cheese, peanut butter, 4 Tbsps. xylitol and heavy cream. Set aside.

Batter:

In a separate large bowl combine water, oil, vinegar, and vanilla. Into wet ingredients SIFT: almond flour, coconut flour, guar gum, xylitol, cocoa, baking soda, and salt. Mix well. Spoon about 2 tsps. of chocolate batter into paper-lined mini muffin baking sheet. Spoon a little peanut butter filling on top. Bake 20 to 22 minutes (yes, they fall in the center). Cool completely. Refrigerate in airtight containers, with layers separated by parchment paper.

Chocolate and peanut butter...
always right.

FACT: *The first recorded mention of the word "cupcake,"*
dates back to 1796, when a recipe notation of,
"a cake to be baked in small cups," was authored by Amelia Simmons,
in the book 'American Cookery.'

CHOCOLATE FACTS:

- The U.S. produces more chocolate than any other country in the world.

- The Swiss eat more chocolate than any other country in the world (in 2nd place is England).

- The Aztecs used cocoa beans as their currency.

- 1.5 billion pounds of milk is used yearly in America to make chocolate.

- The first chocolate bar was made in 1842.

- White chocolate contains NO chocolate.

- 40% of all almonds produced world-wide, go to chocolate making.

- The largest chocolate bar on record, weighed 5,000 pounds.

- Alfred Hitchcock used chocolate syrup as blood, for his famous "shower scene."

LIME-TIME PIE

Crust:
2 cups almond flour
1 cup pecans, chopped
2 Tbsps. coconut flour
⅓ cup butter, softened
1 Tbsp. lime juice
1 tsp. guar gum (pg. 220)
1 Tbsp. xylitol sweetener

Preheat oven to 375 degrees

Mix all ingredients. Press into a deep baking dish (greased with grape seed oil), and slightly up the sides. Bake 15 minutes. Remove, and set aside.

Filling:
5 egg yolks
½ tsp. guar gum (pg. 220)
½ cup lime juice
10 Tbsps. xylitol sweetener
½ tsp. stevia sweetener, powdered
1 cup heavy cream
1 cup coconut milk solids
Refrigerate 1 can of coconut milk, do not shake.
Open can and skim off the solids at the top only.
Use half and half to make up
the difference in volume to meet 1 cup.

Mix all ingredients together. Ladle into baked crust. Bake for 25 minutes. Remove. Allow to cool completely. Cover, and refrigerate.

Topping:
8 oz. cream cheese, softened
2 Tbsps. lime juice
3 Tbsps. xylitol sweetener, finely ground
(in a coffee bean grinder)
2 packets stevia, or truvia, sweetener
2 Tbsps. butter, softened
¾ cup heavy whipping cream
optional: lime zest as a garnish

Using a mixer, whip heavy cream and stevia/truvia to stiff peaks. Set aside. In a separate bowl mix cream cheese, lime juice, xylitol, and butter. Fold whipped cream into cream cheese mixture. Cover, and refrigerate for a few hours. *The longer this sits in the fridge, the better (although overnight will cause it to flatten and get slightly watery)*. Cut pieces of pie to serve. Mix topping before use, placing a dollop onto each slice. Garnish with a little lime zest. Refrigerate leftover pie and topping for the midnight refrigerator run.

Raid the fridge !

A.W.E. – *OMIT lime juice and ADD lemon juice to the crust, filling, and topping*

FACT: *In India, the lime is used to remove and repel evil spirits. For many centuries, it was believed that hanging limes over sick people would cure them of their illnesses.*

CONVERSIONS
3 teaspoons = 1 Tablespoon
2 Tbsps. = ⅛ cup
4 Tablespoons = ¼ cup
8 Tablespoons = ½ cup
1 cup = ½ pint
2 cups = 1 pint
2 pints = 1 quart
2 quarts = ½ gallon
4 quarts = 1 gallon

GIBBLES
(Chocolate-Covered Coconut Candies)

1 cup coconut cream concentrate
(this is NOT cream of coconut)
⅓ cup liquid malitol sweetener
1 tsp. vanilla extract
1-½ cups unsweetened coconut, shredded
½ tsp. guar gum (pg. 220)
½ tsp. stevia
½ tsp. coconut extract
4 bars malitol-sweetened chocolate (pg. 219)
2 parchment lined baking sheets

In a medium size bowl mash the cream of coconut with a fork. Add all ingredients (except for chocolate bars). Mix well. Form dough into ½" balls and place on one of the baking sheets. When complete, put baking sheet in refrigerator to chill. Melt chocolate in a double boiler. Remove from heat. Take coconut balls and place 3 or 4 at a time in chocolate. Roll quickly and remove, placing them close together on the second lined baking sheet. Once complete, refrigerate until solid. Store in an airtight container, in layers, divided by parchment paper. *This recipe yields approximately 140 pieces of candy.*

Mounds of enjoyment.

A.W.E. – *insert half of an almond into a small coconut ball,*
before dipping in chocolate

FACT: *Coconut Cream Concentrate*
(or Coconut Cream as it may be referred to),
is not the same thing as cream of coconut
(the can people are familiar with, that is added to frozen, sweet drinks).

BUDDIES
(Chocolate-Covered Peanut Butter Poppers)

1-½ cups smooth peanut butter (no sugar added)
Sweetener of preference
4 malitol-sweetened chocolate bars (pg. 219)
(in any combination of milk or dark chocolate)
2 parchment lined baking sheets

Pour off, and reserve all the oil from the jar of peanut butter. Place peanut butter in a small bowl. Mix a little sweetener of choice into peanut butter, until you
are satisfied with the taste. (Do not make the peanut butter overly sweet, as the
chocolate on the outside will influence the final result.) Add oil back, 1 tsp. at a
time, until mixture holds together but isn't overly wet. Cover and refrigerate 30
minutes. Remove chilled peanut butter and form into small balls. Dampen your
hands to keep dough from sticking to them. Place balls onto one of the parchment
lined baking sheets, and place them back in the refrigerator. Place chocolate bars
into a double boiler over medium-low heat. Once melted remove double boiler to
a heat resistant surface. Take peanut butter balls from refrigerator. Using a spoon
place one ball at a time into chocolate, and quickly roll it until coated. Place
chocolate-dipped peanut butter balls onto a 2nd lined baking sheet. Work quickly.
If peanut butter balls come to temperature too quickly and seem to be melting
before being immersed in chocolate, place them back into refrigerator to chill.
Once complete, chill the chocolate dipped balls for an hour. Store stacked in an
airtight container, layers separated by parchment paper.

Take one down, and pass it around...

A.W.E. – *OMIT creamy peanut butter*
and ADD your favorite chunky nut butter

FACT: *In the U.S., peanuts account for two-thirds of all snack nuts consumed.*

"FAUX" FRIED ICE CREAM

Dry ingredients:
½ cup pecans, chopped finely and toasted
½ cup pecans, chopped coarsely and toasted
½ cup unsweetened coconut, flaked finely and toasted
½ cup unsweetened coconut, flaked coarsely and toasted
4 - 8 oz. scoops (or 6 - 6oz. scoops) of vanilla or chocolate ice cream
1-½ Tbsps. liquid malitol sweetener
1-½ Tbsps. water
⅛ tsp. stevia sweetener
4 Tbsps. Nature's Hollow sugar-free honey, warmed

*note: Make your own xylitol sweetened ice creams

Preheat oven to 350 degrees

Form ice cream into balls, and place in a freezer container, allowing them to refreeze for 2 hours. Using two separate, parchment-lined cookie sheets, bake the coconut, and pecans *(they cook at different rates, so they cannot go on the same cookie sheet)*. Remove coconut when lightly brown, about 4 to 5 minutes, and sprinkle with half of the stevia when warm. Bake chopped pecans for 7 minutes. Remove the re-frozen, shaped ice cream balls from the freezer. Hold ice cream in your hands for a few seconds, until the outside is "wet," and immediately roll it in the nut/coconut mixture. Place back into the freezer container and refreeze for 3 hours. Combine the liquid malitol and, and place in a small bowl big enough to fit the ice cream balls. Remove the ice cream balls, and roll them in the liquid sweetener, coating all sides. Once again, roll the ice cream into the nut/coconut mixture, and place in serving bowl. Drizzle 1 Tbsp. sugar-free honey (slightly heated), over the top of each scoop. Serve immediately.

I scream! You scream!
We "faux" fry our ice cream!

A.W.E. – *OMIT pecans and ADD toasted, chopped almonds, or walnuts*

OR – *OMIT pecans and ADD peanuts, and use a warmed, thinned down peanut butter (no sugar added), as a drizzle instead of sugar-free honey*

FACT: *Coconut meat is high in fiber.*
Coconuts stay fresh for longer periods of time being stored in the refrigerator, and not left on the countertop.

TOP TEN
ICE CREAM FLAVORS

Cookies 'N Cream

Chocolate

Vanilla

Mint Chocolate Chip

Cookie Dough

Chocolate Chip Cookie Dough

Strawberry

Rocky Road

Mint

Butter Pecan

WHIPPIN' GOOD
(Whipped Cream)

*note: advance preparation is suggested

1 cup heavy whipping cream
¼ cup xylitol sweetener, finely ground
(in a coffee bean grinder)
1 tsp. vanilla extract

Make sure cream is chilled. In a large chilled glass mixing bowl, beat whipping cream on high speed until soft peaked. Add vanilla and 1 Tbsp. powdered xylitol, mixing well. Add remaining xylitol, 1 Tbsp. at a time, until all sweetener is fully incorporated, and cream is whipped to stiff peaks. Cover and refrigerate for an hour. The longer it sits, the less crunchy xylitol becomes, however, if it sits too long your stiff-peaked whipped cream will degrade.

Get your finger out of there!

A.W.E. – *OMIT heavy cream and CHILL & ADD a can of coconut milk,*
after you have skimmed-off the solids (from the top of chilled can),
and whipped it until creamy
(adjusting sweetness level to taste)
OR – OMIT xylitol and use stevia sweetener (1 packet),
which will eliminate the "grainy" texture of xylitol if used immediately

FACT: *Whipped Cream is most often sweetened.*
Sometimes, it's flavored with vanilla extract,
in which case it may be called Chantilly Cream.

CREAMIN' CHEESE ICING

1 cup heavy cream
8 oz. cream cheese, softened
1 tsp. vanilla extract
¼ cup xylitol sweetener, finely ground
(in a coffee bean grinder)

In a small mixing bowl, whip chilled heavy cream to stiff peaks. In a separate bowl, beat cream cheese; vanilla, and xylitol until smooth. Fold whipped cream into cream cheese mixture until well combined. Do not over mix. Refrigerate until ready to use. The longer it sits in the fridge, the less crunchy xylitol becomes.

Yes, you may lick the beaters.

A.W.E. – *ADD flaked, unsweetened coconut, your favorite flavor of extract, or a spice such as cinnamon*
OR – ADD a little of your favorite nut butter
OR – ADD a little cocoa & instant coffee dissolved in a little of the heavy cream, plus more sweetener for a mocha taste
OR – use stevia sweetener (1 packet) in place of xylitol

FACT: *Xylitol, when used in "cold" recipes, and not allowed to melt, can be quite "crunchy" unless powdered.*
Liquid stevia or malitol may be used in place of xylitol, at varying amounts, as they do not require the same amounts.

POSH GANACHE

4 oz. unsweetened baking chocolate
1 cup xylitol sweetener
¾ cup heavy cream
½ tsp. vanilla extract

Using a double boiler, melt baking chocolate and add xylitol. Once xylitol is completely melted, whisk in heavy cream (a little at a time), until combined. Remove double boiler from heat and add vanilla. This may be served warm over cake (like Classic Vanillahhh Cake (pg. 196), or stored and chilled in an airtight container, and used as an icing for cakes or cookies. Yields approximately 2 cups of icing/frosting.

Ganache panache.

A.W.E. *– OMIT vanilla extract*
and ADD raspberry extract
OR – orange extract
OR – your favorite extract

FACT: *What's ganache?*
It's an icing, sauce, glaze, or filling,
that is made to be used on top of, or inside of, a dessert.
Most commonly, ganache is made with combinations of
cream and semi-sweetened chocolate.

BUTTER 'N CREAM ICING

6 Tbsps. butter, room temperature
3 Tbsps. liquid malitol sweetener
¾ cup xylitol sweetener, finely ground
(in a coffee grinder)
¼ tsp. vanilla extract
2 Tbsps. heavy cream
¼ cup cocoa powder, unsweetened

In a small bowl, cream butter. Add malitol and xylitol. Mix well. Add vanilla, heavy cream, and cocoa powder. Great on everything- cakes, cupcakes, or cookies. Store extra icing in an airtight container in the fridge.

Easy to make. Easy to eat.

A.W.E. – OMIT vanilla and ADD ¼ tsp. orange *OR* raspberry extract

FACT: *Butter cream may also be called*
butter icing, or mock cream.

RASPBERRY GLAZE

small container raspberries
3 Tbsps. water
¼ cup xylitol sweetener

For a sweeter sauce, increase xylitol as needed

Place raspberries in a small, thick-bottomed saucepan. Mash berries with the back of a fork, or potato masher. Add water and xylitol. Set heat to medium-high. Cook 10 minutes, stirring often. Use warm over a cake (Classic Vanillahhh, pg. 196), or allow to cool, and pour over ice cream, pancakes, or waffles.

No fighting.

A.W.E. – *OMIT raspberries and ADD your favorite berries*
OR – ADD your favorite herb, such as mint
OR – ADD it to a glass of cold whole milk

FACT: *Raspberries come in many colors.*
These colors include:
Red, Black, Purple, Gold, and Yellow.
Raspberries have been crossed with various species
resulting in a number of hybrids such as:
Loganberry, Boysenberry, and Tayberry.

ORANGE-CHOCOLATE DRIZZLE

3 squares of unsweetened baking chocolate
¾ cup water
1-½ Tbsps. butter
¾ cup xylitol sweetener
1-½ Tbsps. truvia sweetener
(or liquid malitol)
1 tsp. orange extract
½ tsp. vanilla extract

Place water with chocolate squares in a double boiler. Stir often until completely melted. Add butter. Once thoroughly incorporated, mix in xylitol, and truvia. Transfer to a small saucepan, and bring to a low boil for 5 minutes, stirring constantly. Remove from heat. Stir in orange, and vanilla extracts. Upon completion, warm sauce is thin. Refrigeration thickens it. Serve warm over cake (Classic Vanillahhh, pg. 196), or drizzled over Whipped Cream (pg. 212) as a garnish. Also great served cold, as an ice cream topper.

Drizzle sizzle.

A.W.E. – *OMIT orange extract completely,
and INCREASE vanilla extract to 1-½ tsps.*
OR – CUT vanilla extract to ¼ tsp., and ADD 1 tsp. peppermint extract
OR – CUT vanilla extract to ¼ tsp., and ADD 1 tsp. raspberry extract

FACT: *Chocolate contains heart-healthy flavonols
that help increase blood flow, lower your risk of developing blood clots,
and lower your blood pressure.*

More Helpful Hints and Ideas

- ***STRESSED*** spelled backwards is DESSERTS. Feel stressed? Treat yourself guilt-free.

- **Edible Flowers**: Add beauty and color to your desserts.

- **BUY YOUR OWN ICE CREAM MAKER**: Having healthy ice cream or frozen yogurt options is great! Ice cream is an awesome dessert all on its own, or used as a garnish on another dessert. Use it in a homemade milk shake. You decide. Yum.

- **PECAN COCONUT Pop 'Ems:** Toast ½ cup pecans, chopped, and ½ cup unsweetened shredded coconut, by baking at 350 degrees (coconut about 4 minutes, pecans 7 minutes). Melt two bars of chocolate (pg. 219) in a double boiler. Remove from heat. Add toasted nuts and coconut, mixing well. Drop onto parchment lined baking sheet in small bite-size spoonfuls. Chill until solid. Keep in airtight container refrigerated, with layers of parchment paper separating them.

- **FRESH COCONUT:** Once a crack appears in the inner shell of a coconut it develops mold very quickly. You can see mold as yellow, or brown coloring in the meat itself, and sometimes by smelling the shell before opening it. "Wet," or "white" patches in the "eyes" of a coconut, may also be signs of mold.

- **"Cookies are made of butter and love."** Norwegian Proverb.

- **Get more from your eggs**: Store your eggs upside down (fat end up) to extend their shelf life.

- **Substitutions**:
  Don't have 1 cup buttermilk? You can use 1 Tbsp. fresh lemon juice with the remaining volume being whole milk to equal 1 cup. Allow to stand 5 minutes before using in a recipe.

  Don't have 1 cup of heavy cream? You can use ¾ cup of whole milk mixed with ⅓ cup of softened butter, mixing well before use.

"GO-TO" GUIDE

READ. READ. READ.

Become a LABEL reader. This way of eating for health, is based on low-glycemic eating, and the elimination of as MANY TOXINS as possible from your food. When you eliminate Flours, Sugars, Chemical Sweeteners, Soy and Soy Products from your daily diet, you eliminate MOST processed foods.

THE WHY's:

Why is low-glycemic eating important? High insulin levels damage ALL cells in the body. Cell disruption can be the catalyst for ill health. Elimination of foods that spike blood sugar levels (even if temporarily), is important for all people, not just diabetics. This includes eliminating GRAINS (all flours (other than nut), rice, pasta, and breads including what people refer to as healthier "whole" grains), REFINED SUGARS (sugar, molasses, organic sugar, high-fructose corn syrup (HFCS), honey, brown sugar, dextrose, maple syrup, fructose, sucrose, cane juice), ROOT VEGETABLES (potatoes, carrots, parsnips, sweet potatoes (yams) or turnips, etc.), snow peas, peas, and corn. Fruits allowable are berries (in small amounts) and granny smith apples (lowest in sugar). Your holistic healer can supply proper eating suggestions based on your metabolic type.

WATER: We use filtered water because we try to eliminate as many toxins as possible, and this is one of the easiest ways. (Good filtration systems can be expensive.)

SALT: We use Fine Sea Salt and not iodized table salt to limit iodine consumption.

PEPPER: We use freshly ground black pepper for its flavor (or white pepper for aesthetics).

COCONUT: We use unsweetened varieties to eliminate sugar consumption.

COCOA: We use unsweetened cocoa powder to avoid sugar. Cocoa isn't bad for you, sugar is.

CHOCOLATE BARS: (milk or dark): The brand we found is Simply Lite (3.5oz. bars). They do contain some soy lecithin however (GMO source), and should be used sparingly. They are available in milk chocolate, dark chocolate, and dark chocolate with almonds. We also found stevia-sweetened chocolate bars made by Dante Confections, but they require additional sweetening. Or try using unsweetened baker's chocolate, and add the sweetener of your choice (don't be surprised at how much sweetener you need).

BAKING POWDER: We use aluminum-free varieties to limit our exposure to toxins

BACON: We use nitrate-free bacon.

BUTTER: We use organic butter from grass-fed cows, or raw butter when we can get it.

CHICKEN BROTH/STOCK: Organic, no-sugar added boxed varieties, or homemade.

COCONUT OIL: is one of the most stable oils for cooking. Coconut oil requires no refrigeration and may stay fresh for as long as 2 to 3 years. It becomes a liquid when stored or heated above 76 degrees. Unlike other oils, when heated it remains chemically stable and does not create toxic by-products. It only has a moderate smoking point, so cooking with it should remain under 350 degrees (or medium high heat). To melt coconut oil easily for baking requirements, immerse its container in warm water for a few minutes. We suggest you use Virgin Coconut Oil which is minimally processed. It has a mild flavor and smell, unlike Expeller Pressed Coconut Oil which is more highly processed. We use coconut oil, to "grease" our glassware for baking at 350 degrees or lower.

OTHER OIL: Grape Seed Oil (always non-hydrogenated), or Non-Hydrogenated Peanut Oil (most peanut oils are not), should be used at cooking temperatures over 350 degrees (medium high heat). Peanut oil will change the taste of recipes, where grape seed oil will not. However, heating ANY oil to high temperature, will change their molecular structure, thus, making them toxic. Your rendered, nitrate-free bacon fat, is a great alternative for some recipes. *At the very least,* for high temperature cooking, START with an oil that is non-hydrogenated to lessen toxic exposure. Olive oil should be used on cold preparations only.

GUAR GUM is a binding agent and volume enhancer used in gluten-free baking. It has 8x the thickening power of cornstarch. Guar gum is made from the guar bean. It appears as a coarse or finely ground, off-white powder. Use about ½ tsp. per cup of nut flours for baking. In the absence of gluten, guar gum binds baked goods together.

SWEETENERS:

- The sweetener **Xylitol** is a natural occurring sweetener found in raspberries, corn, plums, strawberries, mushrooms and endive, and our preferred choice for baking. It is substituted 1:1 in recipes for sugar. Although it is made commercially, it is considered natural because it is identical to the naturally occurring substance. Since most sugar is made from the cheaper source of corn (rather than cane), xylitol is considered a byproduct of sugar production from corn, and should be suspect for G.M.O.'s. Xylitol is available made from birch trees. It's just harder to find. Xylitol is a low-glycemic sweetener. Overconsumption of xylitol may have a laxative effect, which disappears quickly. The ASPCA considers Xylitol a toxic risk to dogs from lowered glucose levels. *Note: If powdered xylitol is called for in a recipe, rather than spending more money for the powdered variety, simply pulse regular xylitol granules in a coffee bean grinder, a little at a time, to achieve the needed result.* Look on-line for bulk purchasing of sweeteners, your savings may prove to be significant.

- The sweetener **Stevia**, is a plant extract that has 1000x the sweetening capability of sugar. A little goes a long way. It requires more effort to bake with it, as volumes are extremely different. Many people find an aftertaste unappealing. Taste *does* differ between brands, try a few before you make a decision for life.

- The Brand name **NATURE's HOLLOW** makes Sugar-free (all made with xylitol) versions of: Maple Syrup, Honey, Raspberry Syrup, and Ketchup- as well as other products..

- The sweetener **Agave Nectar** is also plant based, but extremely chemically processed. It has a vast appeal as a "honey" replacement, but is high on the glycemic index. We recommend avoiding Agave. **Honey** itself, is also extremely high on the glycemic scale, and should be avoided

- Other sweeteners: **Erythritol, Malitol** may also be used. Note that Malitol is higher in carbohydrates. **Granulated Coconut Nectar** may also be used as a brown sugar substitute, but it has a high glycemic index, as not recommended on a consistent basis. **Truvia** brand is sold commercially, and is a combination of stevia and erythritol.

ALLERGIES: Did you know that a child or adult's "allergy" to certain foods (or food groups), is an "outward" sign of an "inward" problem? Systemic complications from vaccinations, infections, medications, and even physical or emotional stress, may appear as allergies. Your holistic healer can test for, and explain, any and all of these sensitivities to you.

A person that suffers with mold "sensitivities," more than likely has a fungal problem as their primary issue. The foods that people with fungal/mold issues should avoid include, but are not limited to: peanuts, vinegars, ground pepper, aged cheeses (including any variety of blue cheese), mushrooms, and soy sauce. Your holistic healer can guide you, and offer treatment options for these issues.

THINGS TO DO:

- **ELIMINATE SOY:** in all forms when possible including: soybeans, soy lecithin, soy milk, tofu, and soybean oil. Soy Sauce is considered to be relatively safe, as it has been fermented, but it does contain wheat. Use wheat-free varieties to avoid gluten. It is also preferable to use non-U.S. brands, to avoid G.M.O.'s.

- **ELIMINATE CAFFEINE:** as it disrupts your adrenal hormones. Drink weak coffee or tea only if you need to. We would suggest that you use only water-decaffeinated, not chemically-decaffeinated varieties.

- **BUY ORGANIC EVERYTHING:** Remember you are TRYING to eliminate toxins where possible. With regards to proteins (grass-fed meat, raw milk, cheeses, and free range eggs), buying organic when possible will allow you to lower the grain, antibiotic, pesticide, herbicide, fertilizer, and growth hormone influences in your food.

- **ALWAYS WASH fruits and vegetables** well (allowing them to soak in equal parts vinegar and cold water for 10 to 15 minutes) before use. Peel and remove outer leaves (if applicable) before eating or cooking them. Avoid bruised fruits, as they may have larger concentrations of pesticides deep within them.

- Discuss the importance of purchasing **high quality supplements** with your holistic healer. Don't simply purchase what's "on-sale" at your local drugstore.

- **AVOID ALUMINUM AND METAL COOKWARE:** We choose enamel coated cast iron or ceramic pots for stove top cooking, and glass or parchment lined metal pans, dishes, or cookie sheets for baking. No direct contact of food to metals of any kind. We don't even cover or wrap food in aluminum foil, we line it with parchment paper. (FYI: consider removing aluminum based deodorants and antiperspirants, as aluminum is highly suspect, as one of the leading culprits behind Alzheimer's disease.)

- **AVOID CHEMICAL SWEETENERS:** of ALL types -as well as any food containing them, even the most "common" and "popular" ones. They all represent toxins that cause additional health problems in your body. They have been attributed to seizures, memory-loss, increased appetite, the list is rather endless. We encourage you to read up on these, or discuss their toxicity further with your holistic healer.

KNOWLEDGE CLOSET: *(A good reading list for knowledge-cravers.)*

- *The Whole Soy Story,* Kaayla Daniels, Ph.D., CNN

- *The 30 Day Low-Carb Solution,* Dr. Michael Eades, Dr. Mary Dan Eades

- *Knockout, Interviews with Doctors who are curing cancer and how to prevent getting it in the first place,* Suzanne Somers

- *Outsmart Your Cancer, Alternative Non-Toxic Treatments That Work,* Tanya Harter Pierce, M.A., MFCC

- *Heart Frauds, Uncovering the Biggest Health Scam In History,* Charles T. McGee, M.D.

- *Lipitor Thief of Memory, Statin Drugs and the Misguided War on Cholesterol,* Dr. Duane Graveline, M.D.

- *The Great Cholesterol Con, Why everything you've been told about cholesterol, diet and heart disease is wrong,* Anthony Colpo

- *Power vs. Force,* Dr. David R. Hawkins

- *Modern Medical Myths,* Joel M. Kauffman, Ph.D.

- *The Great Health Heist,* Paul J. Rosen

- *The Confessions of a Medical Heretic*, Dr. Robert S. Mendelsohn

- *Lick The Sugar Habit,* Nancy Appleton, Ph.D. (www.nancyappleton.com)

- *Questioning Chemotherapy*, Ralph Moss, Ph.D.

- *The Moss Report:* Ralph Moss, Ph.D., is available for a fee, are individualized reports for people questioning or considering the effectiveness of traditional medical approaches to fighting their cancer. (internet search)

- *The Paleo Solution, The Original Human Diet*, Robb Wolf

- *The No-Grain Diet,* Dr. Joseph Mercola

- *Healing Multiple Sclerosis,* Ann Boroch

- *Wheat Belly,* William Davis, MD

- *Grain Brain,* Dr. David Perlmutter (www.drperlmutter.com)

WEBSITE SEEKERS:

- **www.mercola.com** - Dr. Joseph Mercola operates one of the top-rated holistic websites in the world. He sells high quality products, and hosts a library of articles written by physicians and researchers, regarding the impact of nutrition and toxins, and their effect on our bodies. A truly great resource.

- **www.ppnf.org** - Price-Pottenger Nutrition Foundation offers information on the origins of health through nutrition.

- **www.drronrosedale.com** - Dr. Ron Rosedale, one of the leading authorities on low-glycemic eating, and the publisher of many books.

- **www.jayrobb.com** - Jay Robb offers commercially sold protein shakes and bars that have NO chemical sweeteners, although they DO contain low amounts of soy in the form of lecithin. If you think your protein bar is good for you...read the label closely, and be on the lookout for ingredients under "other" names. Almost all of them have sucralose, or aspartame as sweeteners.

- **www.cwrenviro.com** - A great resource for high quality water filtering systems for shower, kitchen, and whole-house use.

We are glad that you have chosen the path to wellness. We hope to encourage you, as you learn to maneuver through the making of different food choices, in order to support your body on the road to health. This is an exciting time in your life, and we're glad to be part of it.

Daily posts for general knowledge & recipe ideas, may be found on:
FACEBOOK, TWITTER or PINTEREST at **NOW HEAL THIS**

Visit our website at 2wellnessnow.com
for recipe ideas, testimonials, and other information,
to help guide you through a
grain-free, gluten-free, and sugar-free lifestyle.

*Our holistic healer, Dr. Michael Balas, D.C., B.A.,
has an office located in North Bellmore, New York.
He may be reached at (516) 404-7258.*

TESTIMONIALS

Dr. Steve Maraboli, *Author & Behavioral Specialist*

"From delicious healthy recipes, to important facts about nutrition, this delightful book
is a must-have in all households."

Alexandra Martinez, *Writer/Blogger for TLC's Parentables.com*

"*Now Heal This*, has ended the battle between choosing to feed your family good food
and "good for you" food.
Now you can have both –
and a slice of gluten-free, grain-free, sugar-free cake, too!"

Dr. Michael Balas, *D.C., B.A.*

"As a holistic medical practitioner for over 28 years, I am fully aware of the positive
impact a low-glycemic eating plan offers. I recommend it to most of my patients.
Making correct choices in the types of food you consume, plays a huge role in moving
toward maximum health and wellness.
These grain-free, sugar-free, gluten-free recipes
aren't only good for you, but they taste great!
Buy two books.
One for yourself, and one for somebody you love."

Chaplain Jennifer Smith, *Lindenhurst, New York*

"I know God led me to this eating plan, because He knew that 6 weeks later,
I would be diagnosed with breast cancer.
I had already stopped eating grains and sugars, and therefore my body was *really* ready
for the fight of its life.
I went through a mastectomy and reconstruction remarkably well.
I credit God, and the eating plan, for how well I did.
The doctors were amazed at how fast I healed.
I required no further treatment, partly because I stopped feeding the tumors sugar.
Since that time, I have also given up caffeine and artificial sweeteners. I stopped having
chronic yeast and bladder infections. I am more positive and energetic than I have ever
been. I feel great. I don't take any medication.
Eating this way is an easy choice for me. I want to live not only long,
but well, and active! It's been 5 ½ years since I started eating
grain-free, gluten-free, and sugar-free, and I will be eating this way well into my 90's
(fifty years from now). I will still be strong.
Oh, by the way, I'm cancer free!"

Chaplain William Smith, *Lindenhurst, New York*

"I saw myself aging quickly. I was overweight.
I had high blood pressure, arthritis, and asthma.
I started eating grain-free, gluten-free, and sugar-free, shortly after my wife.
I noticed changes almost right away.
I lost weight. I stopped needing my allergy medications.
I had been told by my doctor, that I was on the verge of needing blood pressure
medicine. But, by the time I went back to him for my yearly physical, my blood
pressure was normal. He said to me, "Whatever you are doing, keep doing it."
I no longer have symptoms of arthritis, so I don't need to take all the
over-the-counter pain relievers anymore.
I look 10 years younger than I did 10 years ago.
Completely eliminating grains and sugars from your diet, is something I would highly
recommend to anyone considering their future health."

Ken Mapp, Georgia *(linkedin.com)*

"I have worked with Tina for several years now, and have never felt better, or been
more energetic. I am never hungry, and I eat great!
I am in my early 70's, and taking fewer pills than ever."

Tiffany S., *Bay Shore, New York*

"For 26 years, I have suffered from asthma and allergies.
I was on 7 different medications, and yet I still felt restricted by my asthma.
It wasn't until, only a few months after giving up grains and sugars,
that I was able to stop my medications, and actually enjoy life.
I never imagined there would be a day that I'd be free of asthma!
Another plus...I lost 45 pounds, without exercising.
I love what I eat, and will never go back. This lifestyle change, saved my life!"

Christina Tufano, L.M.T., *Certified Rolfer®, Freeport, New York*
(longislandrolfing.com)

"I am so excited about this cookbook! Tina and Cathleen have been making delicious
recipes for me, for many years. I can't wait for them to share all their secrets. A low-
glycemic, no-grain eating plan, has proven to be the healthiest way for me to eat. *Now
Heal This*, is going to make it even easier for me to continue this eating style, with
wellness as my goal."

Caroline, *multiple sclerosis patient, and poet*

"I wish I had known earlier, how eating changes life-
I would have had less wheelchair time,
less illness, and less strife!"
*note:
As a quadriplegic, unable to move any of her extremities for over ten years, Caroline regained the use of her lower left arm, simply by modifying her diet. She embraced a gluten-free, sugar-free, grain-free lifestyle, and was also able to regain the use of her voice, which for five years prior to her diet change required a voice amplifier.

Big Nick, *Stuart, Florida*

"I am 81 years old. I've had two heart attacks, a stroke, and open heart surgery.
I was a type II Diabetic, with high blood pressure.
When I gave up eating sugars and carbohydrates
(my favorites were bread, pasta, potatoes, saltines, and rice),
I lost 60 pounds, achieving my college weight.
I came off all nine of my medications.
I feel and look younger.
I would tell anyone who is serious about treating any, and all, of their illnesses,
to give up sugars and grains without batting an eye. I did.
My doctors are amazed!
My holistic doctor is expecting even greater things.
You get out of life what you want. Everyone should WANT this!"

INDEX

APPETIZERS

Baked Brie, pg. 87
Bubblin' Crab Dip, pg. 83
Chill-E Crab Dip, pg. 84
Clams Casino, pg. 94
"Cool-As-A- Cucumba" Dip, pg. 92
Devilish Eggs, pg. 79
Eat–Your–Spinach Squares, pg. 88
"Faux" Sushi, pg. 91
Holy Guacamole!, pg. 85
Jalapeño Cheese 'Ems, pg. 89
Let Your Piggy Roll, pg. 86
No-Bones Buffalo Chicken Dip, pg. 80
Party Pleasin' Pinwheels, pg. 95
Pete's Smokin' Fish Dip, pg. 81
Sausage 'N Pepper Pie, pg. 82
Strawberry Salsa, pg. 93
Stuffed "Matoes", pg. 90

BASICS

A Tisket, A Biscuit, pg. 6
Cheddary Bites, pg. 5
Cheese-y Please-y, pg. 12
Chicken Gravy, pg. 18
Churri-Slurri, pg. 16
Cucumber Yogurt Sauce, pg. 9
Dippy Fishy, pg. 10
"Faux" Brown Sugar, pg. 23
"Faux" Crackers, pg. 4
Granny's Applesauce, pg. 24
Granny's Crannies, pg. 25
Herb Butter, pg. 11
Holler for Hollandaise Sauce, pg. 13
Ketchup, pg. 8
"Matoey" BBQ Sauce, pg. 20
"Mato" Sauce, pg. 21
Mayonnaise, pg. 7

(Basics Continued)

No Skimpin' Shrimpin', pg. 10
Oh, Dough, pg. 26
Parmesan Crispers, pg. 3
Presto Pesto, pg. 17
Roasted Garlic 'N Horseradish Sauce, pg. 14
Romano Rounds, pg. 3
There's 'Shroom for Steak, pg. 15
Toasted Pecan Crust, pg. 27
Vinegary BBQ Sauce, pg. 19
White 'N Fluffy Spread, pg. 22

BEVERAGES

Chocolate Milk, pg. 34
Coconut Water, pg. 32
Coffee, pg. 38
Eggnog, pg. 37
Hail to Kale, pg. 41
Hot Cocoa, pg. 34
Milk, pg. 33
Milkshakes, pg. 33
Slushierrrs, pg. 35
Smoothierrrs, pg. 36
Soda, pg. 40
Tea, pg. 39
Water, Water, Everywhere, pg. 31

DESSERTS

Buddies, pg. 209
Butter 'N Cream Icing, pg. 215
Chillin' Raspberry Cheesecake, pg. 190
Chocolate Dunkin' Cookies, pg. 191
Classic VanillAHHH Cake, pg. 196
Cravin' Chocolate Cupcakes, pg. 204
Crazy for Coconut Cake, pg. 197
Creamin' Cheese Icing, pg. 213
Dad's Great Chocolate Cake, pg. 198
Dad's Greater Chocolate Icing, pg. 198

(DESSERTS Continued)

Eat, Gingerly...Cookies, pg. 193

"Faux" Fried Ice Cream, pg. 210

Gibbles, pg. 208

Lemon-Heaven Bars, pg. 200

Lime-Time Pie, pg. 206

Lovin' Raspberry Cookies, pg. 192

Mini-Razzy Cupcakes, pg. 201

OOOrange Chocolate Dippers, pg. 195

Orange-Chocolate Drizzle, pg. 217

Peanut Butter Fudge Mousse, pg. 189

Peanutty Cookies, pg. 194

Posh Ganache, pg. 214

Put-De-Lime-In-Da-Coconut
　　Cupcakes, pg. 202

Raspberry Glaze, pg. 216

Whippin' Good, pg. 212

ENTREÉS

A Chicken-In-Every-Pot Pie, pg. 162

Avocado Relish Flank Steak, pg. 150

Awesome Osso Bucco, pg. 174

Basil 'N Mint Snapper, pg. 178

Chick 'N Parm, pg. 159

Chicken Olé-Olé, pg. 165

Chicken Saltimbocca, pg. 164

Clams, Mussels & More, pg. 184

Cowboy Chimichurri, pg. 151

Creamy Dilled Salmon, pg. 181

Creamy Herbed Pork Chops, pg. 169

Don't Let Your Meat-Loaf, pg. 155

Garden Herb Lamb Kebabs, pg. 175

Grilled Eggplant Parm, pg. 147

Grilled Lime Shrimp, pg. 183

Grilled Pork with Caper Dressing, pg. 168

Herb-Rubbed Chicken
　　On-The-Bone, pg. 166

Lemon Chicken, pg. 157

Let Your Beef Stew, pg. 156

Mahi's 'N Macadamias, pg. 179

(ENTREÉS Continued)

Make Your Pot-Roast, pg. 152

No Shakin' Just Bakin' Chicken, pg. 158

One Stop, Lamb Chop, pg. 176

Pass The Pulled Pork, Please!, pg. 170

Pizza Pizzazz, pg. 148

Pork Chops 'N Applesauce, pg. 167

Salmon Julienne, pg. 180

Spinach 'N Lamb Stir Fry, pg. 177

Stick 'N Chicken, pg. 160

Taco Wraps, pg. 153

Tenderloins 'N Toppers, pg. 154

Veal Chop, with Olive-Caper
　　Dressing, pg. 172

Veal Meatballs with "Mato" Sauce, pg. 171

Very Crabby Cakes, pg. 182

ON-THE-GO

A & A Chicken Salad, pg. 66

Coconut Shrimp 'N Curry Salad, pg. 67

Cumba-Wich, pg. 68

EATING OUT, pg. 74

"Faux" Nola, pg. 61

"Faux" Nola Bars, pg. 62

Fruit Roll 'Em Ups, pg. 72

Garlicky-'Cado Spread, pg. 69

Go...Nuts, pg. 73

Ham-It-Up Salad, pg. 64

Humpty Dumpty Salad, pg. 63

Lovin' Lobster Salad, pg. 65

Pass the Kale Chips, pg. 71

Rolled 'N Ready Ideas, pg. 70

RISE 'N SHINE

Coconut "Up-'N-Eat-'Em" Pancakes, pg. 45

Cravin' Coffee Cake, pg. 56

Family Style Egg Bake pg. 52

Faux 'Nana Nut Bread, pg. 55

"Mato" 'N Egg Nests, pg. 47

Mini Scramblers, pg. 51

(RISE & SHINE Continued)

Nonnie's Bacon 'N Egg Squares, pg. 53
Pepper 'N Egg Cradles, pg. 50
Sausage Gravy, pg. 54
Very Berry Muffins, pg. 48
Wicked-Good Waffles, pg. 46

SALADS

Avocado Ranch Dressing, pg. 121
B & B Salad, pg. 119
Basic Balsamic Dressing, pg. 123
Berry Goat Cheese Salad, pg. 117
Citrus Herb Salad, pg. 118
Cobb Salad Parfait, pg. 115
Duke's Cuke Salad, pg. 116
Eat-Your-Spinach Salad, pg. 114
"Mato" & Mozzarella Salad, pg. 113
Onion Vinaigrette Dressing, pg. 122
Spin Your Salad, pg. 120

SOUPS

Broccoli-Rabé 'N Sausage Soup, pg. 109
Cheesy Broccoli Soup, pg. 99
Cheesy, Creamy, Zucchini Soup, pg. 108
Creamy Cauliflower Soup, pg. 106
Crowded Clam Soup, pg. 103
Easy Escarole Soup, pg. 100
There's Fun-In-Onion Soup, pg. 107
Mexican Hat Soup, pg. 104
Pot-'O-Veggie Soup, pg. 102
Roasted "Mato" Soup, pg. 101

VEGGIES

Broccoli Cakes, pg. 141
Broccoli Slaw, pg. 137
Cabbage Mash, pg. 139
Cheesy Asparagus, pg. 140
Cheese, Please…Cauliflower, pg. 134
Cream 'N Spinach, pg. 132
D.F.O.'s (Deep Fried Onions), pg. 129

(VEGGIES Continued)

Dilly-Dilly Green Beans, pg. 133
Grilled Veggies, pg. 138
Loaded "Faux Tatoes", pg. 142
No-Doubt Sprouts, pg. 131
Nuts for Kale, pg. 135
Roasted Herb "Matoes", pg. 128
Summer Slaw, pg. 136
Zucchini Boats, pg. 130
Zucchini Mash, pg. 127

ABOUT THE AUTHORS

Tina Ellerby, *Author*

Tina Ellerby, born on Long Island, New York, is married, and currently resides in Stuart, Florida. An avid writer of children's books, she found the deviation to writing this cookbook, a natural one.

Having suffered for most of her adult life with an assortment of medical ailments. Tina was amazed to learn the answers to her healing, were staring her right in the face every day, in the types of food she ate. Through the advice of her holistic healer, she began a grain-free, gluten-free, sugar-free eating plan. Her improvement in health was quickly realized, and the news spread throughout her circle of influence. The realization that her friends were just as eager to find improvement of their own health, inspired her. Tina formed a grain-free, sugar-free eating club, and it didn't take long for the recipe sharing to begin. Her frustration in having to "modify" every recipe, and her desire to support family, friends, and even complete strangers in their pursuit of improved health, was the fire that sparked the writing of this book.

Mrs. Ellerby is an active member and children's teacher at her church, and lives at the forefront of elder-care for her family. Beyond writing, her hobbies include baking, singing, and songwriting.

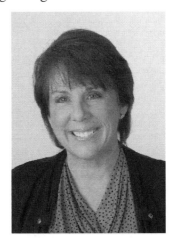

Cathleen Seaquist, *Co-Author*

Cathleen Seaquist, was born on Long Island, New York, and currently resides there with her husband and daughter.

She attended the New York College of Health Professions in Syosset, New York, and became a Licensed Massage Therapist. Certified in many other healing therapies, aromatherapy is where she found her niche. She owns and operates an extremely successful aromatherapy product line. These products are currently sold in many natural organic markets and stores.

Bearing witness to her sister Tina's healing, Cathleen embraced a grain-free, gluten-free and sugar-free eating plan for maintaining her own health. Since she thrives at "blending" natural products for a living, and her passion is to help people, co-authoring this cookbook was a natural progression. She is an accomplished amateur cook, and worked diligently with her sister in the compilation of this book.

Cathleen is an active member of her church, working with children. She enjoys traveling, as well as any opportunity to entertain friends at her home. Her newest joy, is relishing in being a new mommy, and raising a gluten-free, sugar-free, grain-free child.

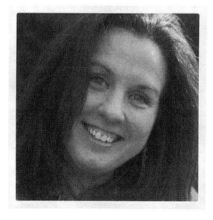

Mommy- kiss God for us.

Made in the USA
Charleston, SC
11 August 2014